Rushing to Yoga

Also by Marilee J. Bresciani

Forthcoming Books:
Surrendering to the Call from Balboa Press

Empowering Leaders out of the Politics of Decision-Making with
Caren Sax from Stylus Publishing

Other Books:
Bresciani, M.J., Gardner, M.M., Hickmott, J. (2009). Demonstrating
student success. Sterling, VA: Stylus Publishing.

Bresciani, M.J., Gardner, M.M., Hickmott, J. (Eds.). (2009). Case
studies in assessing student success. New Directions for Student
Services, 127. Boston, MA: Jossey Bass.

Bresciani, M.J. (ed.) (2007). Good practice case studies for assessing
general education. Boston, MA: Jossey Bass.

Bresciani, M.J. (2006). Outcomes-based academic and co-curricular
program review. Sterling, VA: Stylus Publishing.

Bresciani, M.J., Zelna, C. L., & Anderson, J.A. (2004). Techniques
for assessing student learning and development. Washington D.C.:
NASPA.

For more information, see
http://interwork.sdsu.edu/elip/consultation/index.html

Rushing to Yoga

MARILEE J. BRESCIANI

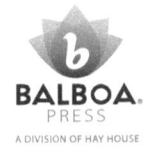

BALBOA.
PRESS
A DIVISION OF HAY HOUSE

Balboa Press books may be ordered through booksellers or by contacting:

Balboa Press
A Division of Hay House
1663 Liberty Drive
Bloomington, IN 47403
www.balboapress.com
1-(877) 407-4847

Because of the dynamic nature of the Internet, any web addresses or links contained in this book may have changed since publication and may no longer be valid. The views expressed in this work are solely those of the author and do not necessarily reflect the views of the publisher, and the publisher hereby disclaims any responsibility for them.

The author of this book does not dispense medical advice or prescribe the use of any technique as a form of treatment for physical, emotional, or medical problems without the advice of a physician, either directly or indirectly. The intent of the author is only to offer information of a general nature to help you in your quest for emotional and spiritual well-being. In the event you use any of the information in this book for yourself, which is your constitutional right, the author and the publisher assume no responsibility for your actions.

Any people depicted in stock imagery provided by Thinkstock are models, and such images are being used for illustrative purposes only.
Certain stock imagery © Thinkstock.

ISBN: 978-1-4525-3472-5 (e)
ISBN: 978-1-4525-3471-8 (sc)
ISBN: 978-1-4525-3473-2 (hc)

Library of Congress Control Number: 2011907343

Printed in the United States of America

Balboa Press rev. date: 6/8/2011

Dedicated to all my teachers, in human form and otherwise, who are walking this path with me, enlightening my every step.

Every day is filled with a multitude of opportunities to exercise choice. In our daily choices, we have the opportunity to advance the power of love. As a result of choosing love, we have the opportunity to feel joy and peace.

CONTENTS

LIST OF ILLUSTRATIONS

The artwork featured on the cover and on the back were photographed by Jamie Gallant in Coronado, California. I am so grateful to Jamie for contributing his time and talent. More of Jamie's photography can be found at www.THEcaskandbarrel.com

ACKNOWLEDGMENTS

I wish to acknowledge with deep gratitude the following beautiful souls for the role they played in the co-creation of this book.

Thank you Cyd, Ralph, Lauren, Elsa, Penny, Kevin, David, Gary, Dan, Danny, Jan, Michal, Mike, Michael, Elizabeth, Cynthia, George, Sharon, Sage, Donna, Jessica, Shaila, Kendra, Peggy, Robert, Dean, Machala, Ixchel, Wayne, Fred, Caren, Sara, Tricia, Sharon, Ruben, Jamie, Chris, Lori, J.D., Irina, Paula, Reo, Ty, and Dad and Mom (although I hope you never read this; you will freak).

I also with to thank the Balboa Press Publishing folks; thank you Valerie Deem, Brandon Drake, Joseph Fatton, Echo Fluharty, Eugene Hopkins, Whitney Johnson, Joan Schaublin, and Rose. I am so grateful to you for all of your patience, coaching, and editing to get this manuscript ready for public presentation.

PREFACE

Engaging in inner work - the work of discovering our authentic selves and discovering the strength to live a life of soul authenticity – is not an easy process. Parker J. Palmer[1] writes "though it [inner work] is a deeply *personal* matter, is not necessarily a *private* matter. Inner work can be helped along in community." Palmer's statement was the motivating force that moved this book to press and encouraged me to begin writing its sequel, "Surrendering to the Call." How did this statement from Parker Palmer do all this?

This book began as an electronic journal. There are many entries in my personal electronic journal that are not in this public book. While, the entries in this book have been dramatized to make a point clearer and while characters' names have been changed to protect their identities as teachers in my life, this book is indeed personal as the events recorded here all occurred in my life. The book reflects the very beginning stage of my commitment to do my inner work. Up until deciding to publish some excerpts of my journal, the journal and thus this book had remained *private*.

A week ago, I was ready to press "send" on the final edited manuscript, approving it to go to press. But then, I stopped. In that moment, I questioned the sanity of making such personal stories public. Why should I make excerpts from my private journal public? Could my academic credibility be undermined by sharing my personal journey to authenticity? Could people use these stories against me in my daily life or my professional life? What if readers don't see the love messages

---

1   Parker J. Palmer (2000). Let Your Life Speak. San Francisco, CA: Jossey Bass Publishing. p. 92.

embedded in each story? What if the stories don't encourage people to practice inquiry in their own lives? What if the stories don't encourage people to practice discovering their authentic loving selves in their day-to-day doings within their own communities?

Questions I thought I had wrestled with and come to terms with weeks before, were now raising their ugly heads once again. The unanswered questions left me sleepless for a week. The morning I read the aforementioned Palmer quote was exactly seven days after I had finished the final edits on the book, yet chosen not to press the send button. I had just been waiting. Waiting for what? I really had no idea. I just knew that I had become afraid to actually publish it. I was afraid of the answers to the questions previously posed. I was afraid to move a portion of my earlier personal life out of privacy.

The morning that I picked up Parker Palmer's book, a gift from a dear colleague and friend, and read the aforementioned quote on page 92 was not a typical morning at all. I was on the Bart, headed to the San Francisco airport to fly home to San Diego. I had been presenting my research at a conference the afternoon prior. The Bart rail system had some technical difficulties that morning, so I found myself with more time on my hands than previously thought for the train was literally stalled on the tracks. Thus, I reached for my hand-written journal to record the dream that I had the night prior.

The night prior, I dreamt that I had flown into some unfamiliar airport. *I had landed safely and gotten off the plane just fine. I had my usual red carry-on roller bag with me, pulling it behind me with my right hand while my briefcase was flung over my left shoulder. I knew I didn't need to go to baggage claim for anything other than to meet the person I had flown to wherever-I-was to meet. In my dream, I didn't know who I was meeting or why but I felt the intense sense that it was very important that I meet with this person and be on time. So I made my way for baggage claim without any hesitation.*

The problem was I couldn't find baggage claim. It wasn't where I thought it would be or where I thought it should be. There were no signs directing me to baggage claim either. I asked several people and each one sent me in a different direction. I wasn't going round and round in circles; I just kept going off in opposite directions, never finding baggage claim but always finding someone else at the end of each route who was very delightful. That person would direct me onto the next route. And each route never got me to where I thought I had to go. I felt growing frustration and increasing anxiety, when all of a sudden I pushed open a door and found myself... outside of the terminal.

The day was gorgeous. It was sunny and warm and very inviting. Yet, I knew my time was growing short. I had to get to baggage claim and meet the person I was supposed to meet. I had to get back in the terminal. The door I had come out of would not let me re-enter. So I headed up a hill on a very wide sidewalk, to go around the terminal where I thought there was another door. On my way up the hill, I thought I saw a swarm of gnats in front of me. I knew there was no way around the gnats for the swarm was simply too large. I had to walk through them to get to the next set of doors. So, I put my head down, closed my eyes, and charged right into the swarm.

Once inside the swarm, the ugly realization for me next was that these flying bugs were not gnats. I don't know what they were but they were biting me and trying to burrow into my skin. Without losing a step, I dropped the handle of my roller bag, flung my briefcase aside and began to peel off a layer of my clothing that the whatever-they-were-bugs were burrowing through. In my dream, I knew better than to open my eyes or lift my head or stop. So, I just kept walking. Peeling off the layer of clothes was not enough however; the nasty little things were now trying to burrow into my skin. I also had to peel off a layer of my skin. I did so with the ease of pulling a tight fitting turtleneck sweater over my head. It didn't hurt; it just felt like the necessary thing to do.

With the laying down of a layer of skin at my feet, I emerged from the cloud of flying whatever-they-were-bugs and arrived at the top of the hill. There, I was greeted by a charming, rotund, elderly, African American gentleman. He was so full of peace and love, I felt rejuvenated from my harrowing adventure upon the sight of him. I asked him where baggage claim was and he began to laugh, a kind of warm and gentle laugh.

"My dear, you walked right by the entrance to it back over there." He was pointing back to the cloud of flying whatever-they-were-bugs. I didn't see the entrance, but I saw my roller bag amidst a cloud of flying bugs.

I looked back at him with anguish. I knew that if I were to try to go to baggage claim now, I would have to go back through the infestation. I wasn't sure what that would mean for me having one less layer of clothing and one less layer of skin. I was aware that I had left my roller bag back inside the infestation, but somehow my briefcase had appeared back on my left shoulder. His peaceful, loving, and joy-filled facial gestures didn't flinch even though I know he could see the pain and anguish on my face. He spoke again softly, lightly, and joyfully.

"My dear, it seems to me that you have two choices. You can either walk back the way you came keeping your eyes open and your head up so that you don't miss the entrance to the baggage claim. Or, you can walk on down that way," he chuckled pointing toward the opposite direction from where I had come, "without your baggage."

I turned away from the gentle man trembling with anxiety and fear. Looking in both directions, I saw the angry swarm and my red roller bag standing amidst it, handle still up, calling me to come rescue it. I looked the other way. I couldn't see anything. The sidewalk seemed to disappear only a few short feet in that direction. I had no idea what to do but the gentle man's words were ringing in my ears. "My dear, it seems to me that you have two choices. You can either walk back the way you came keeping your eyes open and your head up so that you don't miss the entrance to the baggage claim. Or, you can walk on down that way without your baggage."

I spun around to ask the gentle warm and peaceful man more questions; I wanted more guidance. But he was not there. He was nowhere to be seen. I cried out in despair and I awoke.

That morning, the morning after this dream, the moment after I recorded this dream in my journal, I had no intentions of reading the Palmer book. I only had it with me because I had left it in my suitcase from a previous visit. I had just finishing reading this passage ("Though it [inner work] is a deeply *personal* matter, is not necessarily a *private* matter. Inner work can be helped along in community" [2]) when I felt compelled to grab my journal and pen again to re-read the dream I had just recorded.

---

2   Parker J. Palmer (2000). Let Your Life Speak. San Francisco, CA: Jossey Bass Publishing. p. 92.

"Is that a travel journal?" The voice behind me and across the aisle beckoned. I wasn't sure whether I should turn around. After all, I was on a train that was stuck in a tunnel. I just wasn't sure what I would find, especially the morning after the night of a very odd dream. So, I answered as politely as I could without turning around.

"No; this is not a travel journal."

"Are your recording your dreams?" The voice from across the aisle and behind me spoke again.

OK, this can't get any weirder, I am turning around. I slowly twisted my neck and then my shoulders to see the body that occupied the voice that was clearly intent on having a conversation. He was two rows behind me and seated across the aisle. *There was no way he could see what I was actually writing.*

"Yes, yes, it is a journal where I record my dreams." I responded carefully and slowly as I turned. Behind, yet across from me sat a very regular looking young man with sparkling eyes and a dazzling smile. He was full of energy and personality and his effervescence was captivating.

"I record my dreams as well." He responded. "And I re-read them. Sometimes, they read like it was a hangover dream. Other times they make sense to me in a way where I find creative direction in my life." He continued while my mouth was, I am pretty sure, hanging wide open. "When my dreams don't make sense, I share them with my community. They help me discover my creative path." He smiled innocently and triumphantly. I just continued to stare at him, I am confident my mouth was still hanging open. He was not dissuaded.

"My name is Sage." He announced as he scooted up a row and thrust out his hand toward me. He was now one row behind me and still across the aisle. He didn't seem like he was going to attack me, even though I wasn't' sure if he was all there. So, I responded with a smile as his name finally landed on my brain.

"Your name is Sage?" I inquired, reaching out my hand in return, too delighted to really believe that I had just meant someone whose name is Sage who guessed that I was recording a dream in my journal.

"Yes," he responded as he handed me his business card. I glanced down at his card and rubbed my thumbs across it several times as if for some sort of good luck measure. *Yup, his name is Sage and he writes children's books and movie scripts.*

"Of course your name is Sage." I replied still staring at his business card. That is all I could say apart from a mumbled and ill delivered, "It is nice to meet you."

I glanced back up at him and he continued his monologue until the train was repaired and began to move again. I really have no idea how long of a time passed, but it was long enough to cause me to run to the security line after Bart had finally arrived at the airport, request a cut in front of a bunch of very annoyed peopled who were also in the security line because my flight was taking off in 30 minutes, and then run to the gate where my plane was finishing the boarding process.

Finally in my seat on the plane, I pulled out my journal again, pulled out the Parker Palmer book opening it to page 92, and reflected on my conversation with Sage. The three not-so-coincidental moments came together.

Sage had spoken at great length about his community that mutually supports each other to live their creative authentic selves. His community was comprised of friends, family, and co-workers. And after meeting him, I wondered how many strangers also comprised his community. Sage had shared with me incredibly personal stories and asked me very personal questions. In so doing, one observing all this might think he was barging into my life by sharing his stories or barging into my life by asking me to share my thoughts and adventures. But I didn't feel that way. I felt strangely blessed by this encounter with this very odd and delightfully charming man. And I felt that he had brought insight to me about what Parker J. Palmer meant when he encourages us to do our inner work together as it provides us the opportunity to refrain from deluding ourselves with ways of being where others can help us guide us to a place of truer authenticity. I had left Sage having no doubt that he was living his life in a truly authentic way of being; it was beautiful.

My dream from the night before was now no longer a mystery. In thinking I had to go a certain direction in my life and do so in a hurry, I was asking folks for assistance and it felt that they were sending me in crazy paths only to realize that they must have sent me where they sent me so that I could arrive stripped down, through the storm, leaving my baggage behind with a new and exciting road ahead of me. Yet, one I could not see. Yes, I was ready to go off on a new adventure in new skin, with my baggage left behind in the swarm of burrowing annoyances that had kept me from seeing where I was going all along.

Arriving home from the trip, I opened the manuscript, added this preface and realized that the dream meant I had two choices. I could give into the fears of unanswered questions. Or I could do as Parker Palmer encourages and continue to live out my personal life in community with those who help set me on the straight path; the path of authenticity.

Thus, I share this book with you so that it may encourage you to live your personal life in community with those whom you choose; those who challenge you to be that which you were designed to be and nothing less. For me, that has meant sharing some painful memories that led to glorious lessons. And for me, the compilation of lessons shared with a community of friends allows my community to challenge me in new ways that I share in the next book, entitled *Surrendering to the Call*. I hope you enjoy this read.

Namaste,

Marilee

INTRODUCTION

"Hey, don't you need to be getting to yoga?" Penny asked, contorting her arm to show me the face of her wristwatch. Seated cross-legged in my yoga clothes on a wall on the Pacific Beach boardwalk, I glanced her way and noted the time.

Pausing for a moment, I took a sip of my steaming black cup of coffee before I replied, "No, I will wait and go to a later class. I've decided I'm not rushing to yoga anymore."

Standing on the sidewalk nearby, Kevin nearly choked on his coffee as we all burst into laughter.

"Are you serious?" he asked. "Since when have you decided to stop rushing to yoga? And by the way ..." he announced with his Brooklyn accent getting stronger by the moment, "isn't it some sort of irony that you rush to yoga? Isn't that sort of ... well ... counterproductive?"

Before my mind could fully process Kevin's sobering reality check, Penny chimed in, "That's it! That's the name of your book."

All three of us looked up from our coffee cups, glanced to each other, and then howled some more.

"YES!" I screamed out. "You're right, Penny; that's perfect; a perfect title. I'll get started on actually writing that book now! I'll get started on it right away! Thank you!"

Shaking his head, Kevin looked down at his cup and swirled his coffee. The color didn't change at all since there was no cream or sugar in it. It was just black coffee. I wondered why he even bothered to swirl the cup.

Looking back up at me, he smiled; with a sigh and in a great breath of pause, he stated, "Marilee, you rush to everything. Right now, you are ready to rush back home to get started on writing a book you have been talking about for a year. How is that you are actually going to stop rushing to yoga?"

I looked at him with an intense gaze unmatched so far in my life. The smile left my face. I turned my somber expression toward the ocean. The wind, which wasn't present before, caught my hair, whipping my bangs into my eyes. My eyes began to tear, and I couldn't tell if it was from emotion evoked by Kevin's words or from the wind, which was growing stronger by the moment.

Wind: cleansing, yet stinging, something that can't be ignored. The strength of it pulls you from your thoughts as you cling to an umbrella, or your skirt, or your coat ends.

Wind: stings your eyes, as it whips your hair into your face or stirs up the ground around you.

Wind: similar to the pain of truth which smacks you upside the head.

In this case, the bringer of truth was Kevin. As loving as I knew he was in this moment; he was the bringer of truth to my announcement that I planned to no longer rush to yoga.

The following week, not even a full seven days following my announcement from my perch at the beach, I was speeding to yoga, screaming profanities at the driver in front of me who was doing nothing wrong, other than actually driving the speed limit. I cut somebody off—no idea who, nor did I notice what vehicle they drove. I grabbed the recently vacated parking space that they obviously intended to be their own.

Parking is a premium in Hillcrest; there was no way I was going to let an empty spot go, especially when I was running late to yoga. I jumped out of my Wrangler, the most worthy of all vehicles to cut other autos off and make it into tight parking spaces, and threw my bag over my shoulder, knocking the side mirror of the car next to me askew. I saw what I did but I didn't stop to readjust it. I had to move as fast I could to the front door. I had only minutes to spare. *Yes*, I thought as I handed in my check-in card to the gorgeous yoga instructor behind the desk. I had made it; I was in the studio. Now all I needed to do was lay my mat down, change clothes, and I could go through my vinyasas to find that alluring state of peace.

I rushed to the women's locker room and threw my bag to the floor, blocking another yogi's way out of the women's dressing room. I apologized without looking up, and she graciously stood there in complete patience until I noticed that she couldn't step around my bag and me; the changing room was too small. I kicked my bag to the side, still not looking up, and mumbled another apology. *I just have to get into that classroom,* I thought intensely to myself; *then I can become human again.*

Class was awesome; it was just what I had needed; I justified all my preclass insanity for the benefit it had given me. I exited the studio and noticed Vanessa waiting outside.

"Hey you," I called out to her cheerfully, fully refreshed from my renewed spiritual awakening. "Where were you today?"

Vanessa scowled as she replied, "Some asshole business chick cut me off, took my parking space, and I couldn't find another. I didn't want to wait a whole hour and half for the next class but I really need it today."

I stiffened as I heard her reply; the benefits of the yoga class were leaking their way out of my body. I felt frozen in time and space. You know that feeling, that feeling when time and movement freeze as you realize that you have just been embarrassed beyond your wildest imagination. And in your mind, you replay the entire horrible event but you recognize that you can't do anything about it, and since you can't do anything about it, you are now sure that you are going to shrivel up and disappear, or at the very least, pee your pants. But then you realize that time and space really haven't frozen, and now you are staring into space, drooling. And then you recognize that that you haven't shriveled up and disappeared, so now you are really hoping you didn't just pee your pants.

Fortunately for me, my disappearance, or lack thereof, was completely unnoticed by Vanessa. She was wrapped up in retelling the difficulty of not being able to find a parking place and didn't even notice the drool making its way down the right side of my chin. I quickly wiped away my drool as my evil twin began to reason in my head. *She doesn't know it was you who cut her off; don't tell her. I mean, she has never seen you NOT in your yoga clothes with your huge head of hair tightly pulled into a bun. She thinks some bitchy business chick cut her off. You didn't shower; you didn't put your suit back on, she will never know it was you.*

"Uh, Vanessa," clearly the opposite of the devil side of me was about to speak, "I think I owe you an apology."

Vanessa, more irritated by me having interrupted her story, paused for a moment. Then she said inquisitively, "What do you mean?"

"It was m-m-me who cut you off," I stuttered, trying to explain. Vanessa held up her hand to stop me. I thought, *Oh shit, I am so going to get thrown out of this studio for having cut out a fellow yogi from her parking space.*

Before I could think through all my alternative retorts, Vanessa shook her hand in front of me as she exclaimed, "You? You drive a Jaguar?"

"Huh? A what?" I replied with great bewilderment, shaken from the thoughts in my mind of what yoga studio I would attend after I got tossed out of this one.

"You? You drive a Jaguar?" Vanessa repeated, now with some amusement.

"Me?" I responded again, shaken into reality. "Hell no, I can't afford a Jag; I'm a poor college professor. That beat-up Wrangler over there is mine." With that, we both laughed so hard we fell forward, bent over, grabbing our bellies. As we slowly regained our composure and stood upright, we entertained the wonder of who exactly it was that I cut off and who the bitch was who cut her off.

As our laughter died down, I confessed, "Seriously, Vanessa, I got to quit rushing to yoga. I got to start living my life differently." I then told her the story of chatting with Kevin and Penny and Penny's coming up with the new book title. She smiled and put her arm around me.

"I don't know what your book is about, but if you want to interview me for some stories about rushing to yoga, I have some."

"You do?" I replied enthusiastically, wondering where I could quickly grab a pen and paper.

"Yeah," she said, "and you can interview me sometime when I have more time, but to give you a tease, there was one time when I rear-ended a guy, threw my card with my contact information on it out the window to him, and yelled to him as I drove by that I didn't have time to stop as I had to get to yoga. Funny," she said, reflecting, "I never did hear from him." Her eyes perked back up with renewed amusement, as she shared more, "Then, there was another time when I was biking to yoga and a car hit me. I did a fabulous end-over, broke my arm, but I jumped back up on my bike and made it to yoga." She looked at me with pure joy and satisfaction in her eyes. "I did the entire class with a broken arm." Then her cheerful gaze broke. "I got to get to class. We can schedule that interview later."

As I watched Vanessa spring off to the next yoga class, I giggled a while longer. As quickly as the laughter had come with Vanessa, it faded and soberness returned. *I really have to quit rushing to yoga,* I thought to myself, my head hung low in defeat as I walked slowly back to my Wrangler. *I really have to get some things figured out, or one day, I am going to have a heart attack as I rush to yoga. I really have to find a way to live life differently. This way? This just isn't working.*

I started on this book almost three months after my encounter with Vanessa. Four years later, I realized, as I finished it, I never did get to interview her. We were both running too fast and too much. And now, I have no idea where she is. I don't see her at the yoga studio anymore. And I misplaced her business card.

This book is my therapy; it is based on real stories about my life, stories that are not unlike what many middle class Americans may have experienced as they search for meaning. I share these dramatized stories, couched in humor, with the intent that they will inspire reflection and discourse. There are no answers in this book. Rather, I hope the readers will find humor in their own adversities and use them as opportunities to reflect upon the lessons learned with their community of friends. In addition, I hope that when adversities are faced with humor, and that when lessons are learned in our daily lives, we will share those lessons with others so that we all can authentically grow together in joy, love, and peace.

The point of this book is that while awakenings may be found in distant countries as we search to find ourselves or find something, whatever it is that we are searching for, they also occur daily in our regular, everyday lives. And we can benefit from these daily awakenings if we only take a moment to stop rushing around and allow the learning, the remembering to occur. This awareness often occurs when we share our stories with our friends and family. We don't need to spend a fortune, as I have done flying to Bali, where all I came back with was amoebic dysentery, or Italy, where at least I brought back some amazing wine. Our awakenings, our remembering can occur right here in our daily lives as long as we have a sense of humor and some fabulous friends to help us identify them and remember them.

This book is organized, or actually, not organized into a series of randomly placed vignettes labeled as chapters. I share these in the hopes that they will stimulate inquiry and conversation into your own spiritual journey. The names have been changed to protect those not willing to be named, those whose names I have forgotten, or those whom I was simply unable to contact for permission to use their names. I am grateful to all those mentioned in this book; they have been more than a reflection of my thoughts, for they have been my master teachers.

The book ends with a final resource chapter that summarizes some of the concepts introduced in this book and provides a list of resources in case the reader wants to learn more about any one particular concept introduced in this book.

I trust you will laugh, cry, and find renewal within community in the stories that unfold in the following pages.

Namaste!

Marilee

1 Life-Changing Moments

Life-changing moments; what are those exactly, anyway?

Do they occur when you are looking death in the eye one moment and realize you are alive in the next?

Do they occur when you commit your life to someone, have a child, or bury a loved one unexpectedly?

Do they happen when you find yourself in a country halfway around the globe from your home and realize that you have no way to communicate with those you love?

Or do they occur when you acknowledge that half of your life is over and you have been spending most of it in a job you love but now are questioning whether you have really helped out anyone at all?

I suspect that all of these apply; all of these instigate life-changing moments. Or are the just slaps in the face, only to be forgotten when you return to the norm of your routine?

One of my life-changing moments occurred when I was in Pohnpei. Pohnpei is a beautiful country with beautiful people. It is, as you can imagine, a country that does not have the material abundance that the United States does. It could certainly be at the top of any vacation destination based on its beauty and the warmth of its residents, but it isn't. I suspect what keeps it from becoming so is the challenge and expense of actually getting there; the middle of the Pacific Ocean is not a quick destination site.

Pohnpei is about the journey, and I don't mean just about the journey of getting there, as illustrated, for example, in the landing of the plane on some island that barely had room for an airstrip while I was en route to Pohnpei. I was completely disrupted from my book reading when I heard the pilot explain that we would be staying on this island, which had no name, for two days until missile testing was complete.

"Missile testing? Are you fucking kidding me?" I yelled out. Now everyone on the plane knew that I was an American. I didn't care. I could not believe that this plane had landed on an island, which had no name, and I would be there for two days while missiles flew over our heads. *This is so NOT how I am going to die*, I exclaimed to myself. It can't be how I die; there is nothing humorous about this. I am supposed to die laughing my ass off; this is so not what I envisioned. My only saving grace was for me to imagine that I was marooned on Gilligan's Island and would soon find the cast and buddy up to them. After all, Thurston Howell the Third traveled with a full bar. And I was going to need that, I thought, to get through this.

The other passengers nonchalantly filed off the plane while I grabbed my carry-ons and stormed my way to the door. I scouted from atop the plane doorway, before descending the rickety stairway on wheels, attempting to find a place where I could possibly secure a hotel room with electricity. There was none in sight. Caving into the increasingly impatient stewardess, I allowed myself to be ushered to the runway with the rest of the *Gilligan's Island* cast. *At least I have all my shit with me*, I thought to myself. Seeing no sign of a hotel or pub, I began to check my stock of Cliff bars to see how long I could survive. I decided, given the necessity of having to share with the two little kids who saw me rifling through my stash of food, I could survive a week on my stockpile, but I had no idea what I would do about water. *Next time*, I convinced myself, *I am packing the water filter*.

Two hours later (which actually did feel like two days, given my anxiety level), we were allowed to reboard.

As I climbed back up the stairs onto the plane with my luggage in tow, I asked the pilot somewhat skeptically, "So, what about those missiles?" He smiled a devilish smile, encouraged me to move quickly, and assured me that he could take off before the firings resumed. *So this is how I die*, I thought to myself again. *Well, at least it is more original than being stranded on an unnamed island in the Pacific.*

We landed safely in Pohnpei hours later, with no missile mishaps. It was early morning. I checked into a rather lovely hotel with electricity and decided to check to make sure that everything actually worked before night fell again. *It is a good thing I packed duct tape*, I thought to myself as I noticed wires hanging out everywhere and the phone laying on the floor in three pieces. Interesting creatures were crawling over the top of it. I had never seen bugs like that before.

Several hours later, I hung up the duct-taped, now in one piece phone that I had been using to call my boyfriend. As I hung up, I realized I had spent almost six hours of my first day in Phonepei trying to get in contact with the world back home. Apart from my morning run, I hadn't taken a moment to look around and experience the culture.

"That will change tomorrow," I announced to myself. "Tomorrow, I experience Pohnpei." As I peered out the window across the lagoon, admiring the incredible view, a feeling of anxiety began to overwhelm me. I had spent six hours trying to access e-mail so that I could get some work done.

I shrugged my shoulders in an effort to rid myself of the increasingly overwhelming feeling that was creeping up my spine. "Damn it!" I cried out. "Just let it go." I paced back and forth, considering another run to rid myself of the anxiety I was feeling. I couldn't get the thought out of my mind that I had literally wasted the day. *Screw it,* I thought. *I really have no idea why I care. Why is it that I have to feel like I have been productive before I can even enjoy myself anyway? And hell, I have all this writing to do and presentations to prepare. Not having e-mail is a blessing.* "Yeah," I announced to my empty room, proceeding to sit down at my laptop.

"We have power; power is good," I said to myself as I fired up the laptop, pulled a file from my pile of writing projects, and glanced down to make sure the duct tape was still holding the power socket together.

I spent the next hour attempting to pound out an article I owed to one of my professional associations. "Pounding it out" is a perfect illustration of how I was attacking the keyboard. My brain was mush. I pushed myself away from the laptop and decided to try eating a half pound of peanut M&Ms for inspiration. Yes, I brought those with me. There was no way in hell I was going to risk being out of chocolate while experiencing my period. That wasn't anything humankind should witness.

When the chocolate didn't help, I went rummaging through my knapsack, trying to find bubble gum. *Damn, I forgot to pack that. What's a girl to do?* I thought. My mind drifted back to the phone call with my boyfriend. I had reached him briefly earlier but he was at work, so I hung up. Then, I had finally gotten through to him at home but he had another call, from the pizza delivery guy, who couldn't find his apartment, so he had to go. I promised him I would call back, but I couldn't establish contact again.

Is that what is bothering you? I thought to myself. *You are sitting in this hotel room at this beautiful destination. You can't get e-mail; the phone barely works; you can't get your brain in gear to work on this article; your boyfriend just chose his pizza delivery guy over a phone call with you.... Hey, did that really just happen?*

Forget it, I said again to myself. *Just let that go too; let it all go, girl.* I slumped into my chair and peered out at the gorgeous view. *Well, at least I could go take a peek. I deserve to take a peak,* I bargained with myself. I walked onto the balcony and leaned over the edge. The water below was camouflaged by trees and shrubs. It would only reveal itself when the sun reached down to kiss it, causing it to blush. *Beautiful,* I thought, *and amazing.*

As I gazed at the shimmering waves being caressed by the breeze, a feeling somewhat like despair washed over me. *Where did that come from?* I thought as I attempted to shrug it off. *How could I be feeling that?* It was as if a spirit that was riding the wind saw my reflection in the water and reached up to speak to me.

"Your despair is of your own creation. You chastise yourself for not being able to work as you would like in this land. While you believe in what you do, you no longer believe in the effectiveness of the system in which you work. And you are here, questioning your purpose of being here, questioning if you really have anything to teach these people. And your usual distraction techniques are not working."

Instead of returning to my laptop to continue working on the article I had begun (which is my usual strategy for dealing with all things sensitive), I listened to the wind repeat its message. "You are questioning the effectiveness of the system within which you reside. You are questioning the reason you are here. You are running in circles, avoiding what you are to learn here. You are afraid to be in silence. We are ready to teach you, but you must be silent. Will you listen?"

The anxiety and despair were replaced by a wash of fear.

"Am I ready to learn this lesson?" I said aloud to the wind I could not see. My answer came from within: *Yes, you must be ready to learn. You must be ready to learn.* A smile came over my face. It was my smile; it gently replaced the fear, anxiety, and despair that only moments before had overwhelmed me. This must be my life-changing moment. I smiled again as I said aloud, "I must be ready to learn. I am ready to learn. Teach me. I am ready to learn to live differently."

Nine months later, I walked into my first ever yoga studio, afraid of being silent and afraid of being alone with my thoughts. But it was time for me to learn to love differently. It was the beginning of a powerful journey.

2 Regaining My Vision

You are right, I thought to myself as I finished the call with my current beau and set my cell phone down on the counter. *I simply am not getting much out of that relationship.* I stared at my Blackberry/cell phone/home phone/e-mail/calendar/basically left brain lying on the pale tile countertop. For a moment, I struggled with the urge to write myself a note to call the contractor and ask again just when the heck he was going to install my new countertop, now that he had my $500 deposit to take a measurement that hadn't even been taken. As I reached for a pen and paper, I began to giggle to myself. I added that I wasn't getting much out of that relationship either. I glanced down at the pen and paper in hand and completely forgot what it was that I was supposed to remind myself to do.

Instead, I moved toward my kitchen bar stool perch, pulled my glass of shiraz closer to me, opened my laptop, and began to write, "After forty-four years and five months, I am turning in my *Lost in Another's Vision* card. Do you hear that, universe? I am no longer going to lose myself in another's vision!"

I laughed aloud as I reached again for my shiraz. Sipping and twirling the deep red liquid, I reflected.

It is true that I find great meaning in helping people discover their talents, in finding new direction for themselves that they find more fulfilling than their current paths. I find satisfaction in facilitating people's connection with their hidden gifts and great fulfillment when I see the light in their eyes sparkle as they discover what a gem they truly are. I love to facilitate others' connections with their dreams. However, I had decided, after forty-four years and five months of my own enlightenment, that I would no longer be at the beck and call of any of the people to which I did this and as a result, lost my own vision; that happened to only apply to those I dated.

I smiled as I pushed the laptop away and reread the words "I will no longer be lost in another's vision" in black and white; the cursor flashing innocently on and off on the screen. Maybe that is what the relationship coaches were trying to teach me. I am such an idiot. Three coaches and $7,000 later, months after at least a dozen girlfriends and guy friends had told me this, I realized that loving someone, helping them realize their dreams, does not mean you need to be at their beck and call. It does not mean you have to lose your own vision.

"Damn it," I exclaimed aloud, startling my reflective mood. "If I had that seven grand back, I could hire a new contractor and possibly get this countertop replaced before another decade passes."

I laughed at my own stupidity. I was grateful for the distraction of the countertop and the humor it provided me. Yet, the distraction would not last. Returning to the memory created by the earlier phone call, my head began to spin as that one memory created a cavalcade of earlier memories, all ironically similar. One love after another, I recalled how in each situation, I neglected my own relationships with others or myself to make sure that the one upon which I was focused knew that I was invested fully in his dreams, in the discovery of his talents, in the encouragement of his gifts, and yes, at each moment when his dream was realized, I departed, not even staying long enough to celebrate his newfound victory with him.

"Now that is a problem," I announced to my empty kitchen, leaning back on the bar stool. "Wouldn't a sane person stay around long enough to reap the benefits of her investment?" I paused, glancing at the orchids, expecting them to answer. When they didn't and all I could hear was the ticking of the clock, reminding me that I had a student's dissertation to read before I could enjoy the comfort of my bed, I leaned forward, pulled my laptop closer, and returned to my electronic journal.

So, I spent the seventh phone call in a row listening to him tell me about his new life now that he is retired, all the things he can try and how I was just the perfect woman to make his dreams come true. Yes, with my encouragement, he could become a millionaire, he could launch the career that he always dreamed of, and I would be key in providing him the emotional support he would need.

The thing is, I liked hearing that. I like being somebody's cheerleader. I like being the one who helps him/her see his/her talent. I don't lie; I don't exaggerate. I just get to see what people are really capable of and then I get to share that with them in a manner they can grasp. But the funny thing is that when I do this with women or men in whom I have no romantic interest, I can share this and back away. I don't lose my own vision or myself in them. If I am attracted to you, well, apparently, I have to become consumed by your dream until the point that all you see is simply your personal muse with no needs of her own. I do it to myself.

"Well, no more," I told my journal.

"No more," I announced to the orchids and to the cracked countertop and to the contractor, which reminded me what I was supposed to write on the pad of paper.

Instead of writing, "Call the contractor," I wrote, "It is possible to love someone or several people, to see their dreams, to identify their talents, to encourage them in achieving their dreams, and to remind them that their consumption of their dream does not mean that they can consume you. For you are gifted and have a vision to fulfill that may not align with theirs. Yes, you can and will be the hero of someone else's passion, but you can also be the hero of your own, if you choose to be. I choose to be the heroine of my own passion, the encourager of my own dreams, the visionary of my own life."

3 Feeling Trapped

I watched her from across the table; my heart was moved beyond measure. Tears were streaming down her lovely young cheeks as she brushed her blonde hair behind her ears. A few strands were caught by the tears on her cheek, and the sight of it pulled at my heartstrings even more. I looked down at my half-eaten salad, hoping she wouldn't notice the need to fight back my own tears. Oh, how my heart ached in empathy for the pain that she was experiencing. Breathing deeply three times, I caught a bit of courage to look back up at her again. The scene had not changed.

"Evelyn," I began with a voice much more courageous than the one I actually felt coming from within. "You are not trapped. You can get out of this situation if you want to do so."

Her right eyebrow rose with curiosity, causing the hair behind her ear to fall in front of her eyes. As she brushed it back again, I noticed that it no longer clung to the tears on her cheek. The sight of it gave rise to a smile on my face, and I continued.

"You are not trapped," I repeated. Feeling the energy of hope emerging from her bosom, I pressed on.

"You can get out of this situation if you so choose." Mutually rejuvenated by these words, I continued.

"Unlike many in this country, you have the personal resources, friends, and family to support you, to get yourself into a place where you can feel safe enough to replenish yourself and then actually think through your options. That is a gift that you have; I recommend you take advantage of it."

Evelyn paused, looked down into her untouched crab cake salad (you should never order crab cakes outside of Maryland; they actually did look inedible), and her soft blonde curls fell again into her face, now once again streaming with tears.

"I am trapped," she cried out. "No one ends a marriage after only one week of being married."

At this point, the counselor side of me (which never existed at any point in my life to begin with and existed even less at this moment) completely subsided.

"Are you fucking kidding me?" I exclaimed, way too loud in the quiet little Italian bistro; heads turned my way in complete and utter disgust. I courteously yet efficiently gave them all a soft *Don't mess with me here, I got issues to deal with* look, which caused them to quickly and submissively return their attention to their own tables.

"Evelyn," I stated strongly with my newfound composure, "did I ever tell you the story of my first marriage?" This comment, so much more than the previous crass one, seemed to pull Evelyn from her own inner world.

"Your first marriage?" she asked, now curious.

"Yeah," I answered in such a matter-of-fact way that only those who have been married more than once can pull off. For the first time that evening, Evelyn now had an expression that was different from sorrow; she seemed almost amused.

"My first marriage ...," I repeated in an attempt to reel in her amusement as if I was playing to a personal audience.

She tilted her head, prepared for the show, her long blonde hair falling to the side of her face as if to pull it even further toward the table.

"Yeah," I repeated, "I felt my first marriage was a failure within the first twenty-four hours. Let me rephrase that," I interrupted my own self with a clearing of my throat. "I *knew* it was a failure within the first twenty-four hours."

Evelyn's head bounced back to life, and the gleam in her eye brought renewed hope to what should have been an awkward and sorrowful conversation.

"Really?" she replied, her head and hair tilting to the other side.

"Really," I stated with full confidence. "And seven years after that first twenty-four hours, he finally filed for divorce."

Her mood changed once again. In an attempt to keep her from the abyss of pain, I continued, "Ego, Evelyn; ego kept me from talking to anyone sooner, from seeking help earlier, from admitting to myself that something was not quite right. Ego, Evelyn; ego set the trap that I fell into, and as a result, I lost seven years of my life; I lost it to the trap of ego. I had family, I had friends, I had financial means to get out of the trap, but I chose to be subservient to my ego instead. Evelyn, often circumstances do not trap us; stupid decisions do not trap us. Our ego traps us; it causes us to think that we can't get out of a stupid decision because we may disappoint another, whomever, or ourselves. I am from a working class family. You are from the upper middle class. We are only trapped as much as our ego or pride allows us to be trapped. Girlfriend, you and I can't even begin to comprehend what 'trapped' really is, so quit telling yourself you are trapped. You are not trapped. Choose to believe you are not trapped."

Evelyn bowed her head, stared at her crumbly crab cake that had way too much stuffing, took another bite, and with her mouth full, promised me she would think about what I had just said.

As I drove home after dropping Evelyn off, I thought about the critters who chew off their legs to get out of a trap set by hunters. In all of the moments that I had felt trapped in my life, I never considered chewing off my leg. I did dream about that knight in shining armor riding up on his white horse to rescue me. I did dream about winning the lottery or simply running away or disappearing. But I never considered chewing off a limb. I guess that meant that the only trap that was set was the one my ego had set for myself. And therefore, I was the only one who could release it. And that seemed equally true for my friend Evelyn.

4   Celebrating Weddings

There is nothing worse for a heartache than going to the wedding of a dear friend. Don't get me wrong, I am not adverse to weddings, especially for people I love dearly and for people I know are making a healthy decision. However, when the guy you have been dating for four years is on vacation with his former wife and two kids (and you aren't invited along) four and a half hours away from where you flew in to see your friend get married, well, focusing on celebrating a wedding is the right thing to do, but finding the strength to do it is nothing short of a challenge.

On this trip, I felt it was going to be easier to do the Marine Corps fitness test than survive this weekend. And in order to honor my dear friends who were getting married, I needed to do more than be on survival mode, I needed to be fully present for them, to honor them and support them on their new journey together. Furthermore, they asked me to sing a song of my choosing during their ceremony; I wanted to do my best!

But that was not what I was thinking as I boarded the plane to the wedding destination. What I was thinking was that I could either bury myself in work on the plane ride or pray that there was enough alcohol on board to place me into a short three-hour coma. As my anxiety arose, I began to lean toward the latter option. Referring back to the Marine Corps fitness test, however, I thought that what I should be doing is drinking plenty of water, getting some rest, and doing some mental preparation/meditation to prepare my body, or in this case my spirit, for what was to come; that would have been the healthier choice. And I was hell-bent on choosing that until *he* joined me in my empty row in the back of the plane.

His name was Jamie. He was the kind of airplane passenger who ignores all the clues that you don't want to chat. He talks loudly while your i-Pod earphones are in your ears, leans over across the papers you are grading to ask what you are reading, and talks to you enthusiastically about what type of Mac you have when it is clear you have the basic of all basic kinds (well, basic for Mac). I even read to him all of my "Conversation Stopper" quotes that are printed on the back of the free drink coupons that Southwest hands out to its frequent fliers. All he did was laugh and ask if I had enough free drink coupons to share with him. I explained to him that given the length of the flight, the fact that he was I was going to a seated next to me, and that wedding, I would be needing the booklet that I was holding in my hand and another booklet of ten, just for myself.

Fully expecting Jamie to now finally get the hint that I was in no mood to chat, I repositioned my laptop and reached down to reconnect my earphones. Ignoring my gestures completely, Jamie burst into laughter and asked me if I would join him in a rum and Coke. I glared at him for a moment, but his smile wouldn't fade. I leaned into the aisle, looking desperately for another free seat; however, the only free seat on the plane appeared to be the one in between Jamie and me. Letting out an exasperated sigh, I shoved my laptop, papers, and i-Pod aside and prepared myself to be fully entertained by him. I gave the attendant two coupons when she passed by and asked her not to stray too far. She smiled understandingly and allowed me to keep one of my two coupons, the one that held the best, yet still ineffective, conversation stopper, which read, "It takes me at least two drinks to be able to talk, and I usually stop talking after the first one."

I read it quietly to myself and then laughed aloud; I turned to Jamie and invited him to tell me his story. Jamie was forty-four and had been married four times. He was not currently married, was still very open to falling in love, and was very confused by my increasing anxiety as the wedding destination approached.

I explained to him that my anxiety was rather complicated. I started with my first point, explaining that I had allowed my two former husbands to break my heart so fully that I saw no point in marriage. Jamie seemed completely confused. Of course you are confused, I thought to myself; we are the same age, and you have been married four times and are clearly inviting number five into your life. Me, on the other hand, I couldn't comprehend the emotional capacity that would be required for two people to stroll up the aisle and declare either that they were not going to change enough to annoy the other greatly or that they would be completely okay with how each one changed and grew.

"Do you know the emotional capacity that is required of a person to enter into marriage?" I exclaimed with way too loud of a voice and way too exaggerated arm motions.

For the first time in the plane ride, Jamie became concerned that our voices were carrying too far and suggested we tone it down. I was shocked by his announcement. While I chose to be respectful and lower my voice, I decided not to let him off the hook. "Well," I exclaimed, this time a little softer but with even more intensity, "do you know anyone who has that kind of emotional capacity?"

He looked down at his rum and Coke, well into his second, while I was still nursing my first glass of wine.

"Do you think you have changed that much?" he replied. "Don't you think you still have the same core values?"

I smiled, as I replied, "Core values? Yes. But I don't express them or live them out now anywhere similar to the way I did at twenty-two, thirty, or even forty. And I like that very much about how I live," I replied.

The smile from his face melted, and I began to feel as if I had just brought Jamie down. Feeling responsible for tearing the smile from his face, I punched him softly in his large muscular shoulder.

"Hey," I said playfully as I punched him again, the way sixth graders flirtingly tap each other when they pass in the school hallway. "Are you okay?"

His faced warmed at my touch, and he looked up from his third, now completely finished rum and Coke.

"I see what you are saying," he said smiling but sounding completely defeated.

Oh man, I thought to myself. *I didn't need to go put my downer mood on anyone else. I should have kept it to myself.* I felt I needed to remedy this moment urgently.

"Listen, my friends who are getting married are in their midfifties. You know what?" I said overly cheerful but expecting that he may not notice. "I bet they will be able to provide each other plenty of space to grow and become who they are while staying happily married. I mean, heck, at some point in life, growth has to slow down, doesn't it? At some point, we should be just fine stating we will be okay with that one person for the rest of our lives."

He smiled, fully "on" to my attempt to cheer him. He retorted playfully with a question back at me: "So, will you stop growing when you hit fifty-five?" I laughed loudly, but this time, my loudness did not seem to bother him.

"Good one, Jamie," I smiled. "I better not remarry until I am eighty-five." With that, we settled into more casual conversation. I giggled when he asked me what my favorite color was. I haven't been asked that since I attempted to date on E-harmony, a process that annoyed me to no end and a topic for a later time.

As we exited the plane, he invited me to his home to water ski the following weekend. Saying that I would consider it as we exchanged business cards, I walked away, knowing full well I would never see him again. After all, my heart belonged to the man who was on vacation with his former wife and kids.

The following day in a gorgeous mountain setting, just outside the "ready room" of the beautiful bride, I stole away for a quiet moment of my own. I reflected on my anxiety about the wedding, just minutes away; I thought of my guy surely tending to his kids at this very moment; I thought of Jamie and the energetic and enthusiastic way he approached love. And in that moment, I chose to place my cynical nature aside; I chose to adopt the innocence of the four-times-married, forty-four-year-old man and engage fully in the wedding of my friend.

Confident in my decision, I looked up from my hiding place toward the bride's room. Before I could move with my newfound plan to fully be present for her, I saw the groom lightly tap on the door. *Oh man, I* thought, *could he be changing his mind at the last minute? If he is, should I tackle him or let the news just fall?*

Before I could decide what to do, I saw my friend push the door open, cracking it slightly and ever so softly. Upon seeing him, she threw it open, her eyes full of light and her face radiant. They looked into each other's eyes, holding hands like two kids ready to play. I couldn't hear what he was saying but I did see the look on both of their faces.

I blinked hard, tears rolling down my cheeks. I didn't even think of how my make-up must be smearing. *Damn, Jamie,* I thought to myself, *this is what you were talking about.* At that moment, I became even more committed to being there for my friend, and I completely forgot about my love not being with me to celebrate this moment, but rather being with his former wife and kids, and I strolled over to the door, playfully chiding the groom for seeing her before the ceremony.

The ceremony was magical, and I sang my song for them without crying. As I stood in the back of the reception, watching couple after couple dance with each other, I thought to myself, I love how the universe intercedes, providing us with distractions just when we think we don't need it. Reflecting back on that conversation with Jamie on the plane, I wondered, *Was he an angel sent to help me through this moment? Or was he real?* Pulling his business card from my wallet, I decided to choose to believe that he was an angel sent to help me move into a better place just so I could fully be there for my beautiful, now married friend.

Placing Jamie's card on the table just next to my glass of unfinished cabernet, I strolled onto the dance floor all by myself, completely forgetting about my love, vacationing with his former wife and kids. I danced to new beginnings and peaceful endings. I danced to renewed hope and never-ending love. I danced to the truth that love never ends, it only changes form, and I danced to those who have the courage to recognize that, to believe in it, and to act on it.

5   Safe and Secure

Wouldn't it be great to feel that feeling again? You know, the one where you feel safe and secure and have no doubt that you will always feel that way? It may have occurred when your dad or mom tucked you into your bed at night. Or perhaps it occurred when you were preparing for a road trip with your beloved. You just knew that all you had to do was get on the road with that person and all would be well; you packed the picnic basket, he had the road trip planned and would be driving; all you had to do was get into the car. You could just sit back and enjoy the scenery. For others, it may be that feeling you get when you settle into first class on a long flight. *Ah,* you say to yourself, *I am here, settled into first class, my drink is on its way, I am buckled in, and the pilot has the helm. My cell phone is shut off, no one can reach me, and I am truly safe and secure.*

Well, I used to know what those feelings felt like. I yearn for them to return, and all I can say now is that there is no such thing as safety or security. Everything—and I mean everything—I used to find safety and security in no longer exits. My favorite blanky has long since been shredded. My trusty driver turns moody and tempestuous after too many hours on the road. And who was the idiot who thought installing Internet on airplanes was a good idea? My savings plan has erupted. Now that I have tenure, the state where I work is bankrupt, so I may not even get paid for the job I earned the pleasure of being able to keep.

Nope, nothing is safe and secure. The only thing we can count on is change; the only thing we can embrace is ambiguity. And even when we count on being able to do that, we grow stagnant and unable to think or create for ourselves.

So, what is the secret to finding safety and security? I discovered it could be found from looking within.

On one particularly bad night, I was in a hotel hallway, just outside my room, sitting on the floor, talking on the phone with the man I love. I was in the hallway because I had just brought my father into the hotel room; he had suffered a heart attack on his way to see my sister. Since I was the one with the most frequent flier miles, I was able to fly back and take my father and mother to the nearest emergency room. Fortunately for all of us, they were in Dallas/Fort Worth and the hospital was Baylor Medical, a wonderful place to be when your father has an emergency and is in need of excellent care.

I am not exactly sure what time of night I was on the phone with the man that I love but it was late, I was tired, and I was emotionally spent. I had spent several days prior fearfully watching my father, the pillar of my life, as we learned just how severe his condition was. I was not ready for my father to be fearful; I was not ready to see him in a place of fear. He was the last remnant of security in my life to which I was clinging, and now, I saw that even that was fading.

As I was desperately trying to explain my emotional state to my love in as calm a voice as possible, it dawned on me, or rather on him, that I was completely falling apart, right there in the Holiday Inn Express hallway in nothing more than my tattered sweat pants and tank top.

As I began to sob uncontrollably, the voice of strength that I so loved came clearly across the phone: "Babe, you're a mess, aren't ya?" Rocket scientist, he is not.

"Well, darlin'," I tried to explain as calmly as possible to keep the "neighbors" from opening their hallway doors to see what sort of entertainment had landed unexpectedly near them, "I guess you could say that. I mean, that is my dad in there and he is my pillar. And now

I feel that my pillar is crumbling, along with everything else. What exactly do you recommend I do about that?"

Before I share with you his response, I need to let you know that I had been dating this man for about four years. However, he wasn't really "available" at that time to date (another story indeed this will be), so I broke it off. However, when he did become available to date, I was "way more into it all" than he was. At the time of this phone conversation, well, I was "way more into the relationship" than he was.

After a short but very dramatic pause on the phone, long enough for me to greet the two very drunk guys getting off the elevator in a manner where I could convince them that I was not their misplaced hooker for the evening, which was extremely difficult to do, given the fact that my belly was showing in my scantily clad evening sweatwear, my love replied, "Well, I recommend you first get off the phone with me. Then, I recommend you do some meditation or yoga if you have enough energy. Then, I suggest you get some sleep so that tomorrow, you have the energy and strength you need to become the pillar that your father and your mother now need."

The phone dropped from my hands. This was not quite the message I was looking for. I was looking for this hot stud of a man on the other end of the line to ride, somehow, across half the country in five minutes, to come rescue me from my pain. I stared at the phone in disbelief, still lying on the hallway hotel carpet. Distracted by a patch of unidentifiable grime that was next to my phone and immediately wondering what the hell kind of grime I was sitting on at the moment, his words caught my attention once again.

"Babe, babe, are you there?"

"Yeah." I stifled a sniffle, as the tears began to flow again. "Yeah, I am here."

"Talk to me," he replied, which was his amazing way at getting me to come back to reality regardless of what planet I managed to drift off to.

"I'm okay," I lied.

Knowing full well my lie, he offered further encouragement and sound advice.

"You are there with your dad and mom, and your family needs you to reach into what they have created inside you; you have the strength of both your father and your mother within you; you have the strength of you and all those who have invested in you right there, right now. I can't be there, babe. So, go refuel yourself and in so doing, go refuel all those who have made you who you are. Tap into that energy, and let it see you through."

I wanted to be angry with him for not being there physically in that moment, even though he had earlier offered to fly to be there with me. Instead, a warmth and energy beyond my recognition swelled in my bosom. My eyes didn't know whether to cry more or smile. This feeling was new to my eyes, and they didn't know how to respond. My long pause drove again his words, "Babe, are you there?"

"Yeah, sexy," I said. The smile that was finding its place on my face caused my eyes to feel as if they were wiping away their own tears. "I am here ... thank you."

A few moments later, after closing our conversation, I rose from the hallway; the tears had dried on my cheeks, and my knees creaked with anger for my obvious neglect of their needs in the way I had crouched in the hallway. I smiled as I glanced down. There was no more grime to be seen. What exactly did I see anyway? It must have been the reflection of my mood and nothing else.

I quietly made my way into the room; I used the light of my cell phone to look upon the faces of my dad and mom; they were sleeping peacefully and apparently quite happily. I sat on the edge of my bed, recalled the prior days, the present day, and the present moment. My eyes chose to respond positively to the smile that once again found its way to my face. I turned off my cell phone and laid back into the comfy bed. *What was that I felt?* I thought as I began to meditate. It was a feeling of safety and security washing over me. *Where did that come from?* I thought again. *It came from within.*

My entire face smiled, as I drifted off to peaceful sleep. Safety and security is not elusive, unless we choose not to seek it from within.

6   The Abyss

I really enjoyed the movie that shares this chapter's title. I loved it; a story of adventure; of mystery; and of hope in some sense. And then just when you thought you were so confused, meaning arose and so did a rescue; an amazing miracle of a rescue that launched into more of a dream, more creativity, more imagination, and more hope.

For some, there is hope in not knowing what lies in the darkness or what lies in the light. When you peer into the abyss, hoping to catch a glimpse of light or some sense of meaning; well, I think that is a hope of all hopes; staring into the darkness of the abyss searching for light, searching for answers, searching for meaning, searching for a renewal in our own beliefs. That is hope.

And so goes my life with the Internet. Quit laughing, I am serious. Consider the Internet the abyss. Really, I am serious. Consider how we search the web trying to find our soul mate, looking for answers to questions or to forecasts of the future. We search for connections to lost loved ones, to current friends and colleagues, and we always, always search for answers to simple questions and to complex ones. The Internet is the abyss.

Consider also how we text a friend and then stare at the screen. We stare into the abyss of light (or darkness, depending on our own personal cell phone settings or mood), waiting for the answer back. We do the same with e-mail. You know, you send someone an e-mail with a question or a witty retort. *I wonder when they will reply*, you ask yourself somewhat impatiently. So you wait, pretending not to do so, looking ever so frequently into your inbox, hoping to see if a reply has come. We are seeking hope in the electronic abyss of the Internet. And I wonder how the answers that we get from it reflect ourselves, our deepest sense of self. I wonder.

And that is my story tonight. I sent my love a text, saying I'd like to fly out and see him this weekend, asking if he had time to talk about it tonight before I headed to bed. I sent my message of hope into the abyss, and I kept looking at the screen, but I saw nothing. I stared into the Internet abyss, hoping to see an enthusiastic response of how he wanted me to fly to see him, hoping he would offer to make the arrangements on his own as I am so busy. I didn't communicate any of this to him; instead, I stared at the screen and hoped.

I looked down again at the dark screen, and my eyes lit with excitement when I saw I had a new message. "Oh man," I cried in a defeated voice. It was a text, not from my love, but from my colleague, letting me know our deadline was growing closer and asking me to answer a question she had. The abyss had sent me back a message, not of hope but of fear.

I looked away, pretending not to read her plea; the flood of all sorts of deadlines came crashing down on my hopes, collapsing my dream of spending the weekend with my love. But no, I couldn't accept the fear and dread that that text brought. I didn't want to face reality again, just like in the movie. I didn't want to suffocate from too much work. I wanted to choose hope. So I dared to glance down again, thinking maybe her text will disappear into the darkness and his will reappear in the light. But nothing had changed. Her text was still there, appearing even brighter, and his was … absent.

I took a deep breath. Once again I looked away from the Internet abyss and gazed at the ceiling. Perhaps a glance toward the heavens would bring the hopeful message from the abyss. I laughed to myself as I thought how silly I must look, and I was grateful that no one could see into my hotel room where I sat all by myself. I continued to stare longingly toward my makeshift sky, and the blinking light of the smoke detector reminded me that maybe I had a message waiting for me, a message of hope from the abyss.

Glancing back down, I paused with my hand hovering over my phone. I knew he hadn't responded. All that awaited me was her text, reminding me of the approaching deadline and the work I had yet to complete. With great courage, I tapped the screen, and it was true, no message from him, just another text from another colleague to whom I owed work.

The abyss had brought me no hope, only the reminder that if I didn't get moving on my workload, I may most assuredly fall into despair. I laughed at my proclivity toward drama as I pushed my cell phone out of my eyesight. I pulled my laptop toward me in its place and resisted every urge to see what my horoscope said might happen today. Instead, I disconnected my wireless access and opened the document I owed my friend.

Glancing back at my cell phone, I resisted the urge to check the Internet abyss one more time and chose, instead, the known of my universe, which was my work. Failing to resist another time, I grabbed my cell phone and hit the button; nothing again. My heart fell as I wondered how many minutes of my life I truly have spent staring into this abyss and others like it, searching for hope, searching for answers, searching for affirmations of love.

My cell phone slid from my hand onto the desk. I pushed my laptop back into its original place. My physical fatigue was telling me that it was time for bed; time for rejuvenation; time for dreams. As I considered my schedule for the next day, I realized that hope would have to come from my dreams instead of the texts from my cell phone; in the restoration of my sleep instead of the unanswered e-mails; and in the sustenance of the glass of water I was now using to wash down my multivitamins instead of the answers I didn't find on the web. As I moved from my desk to my bed, I checked my cell phone once again; two more work texts. My abyss seemed to be growing more dismal.

As I eased into bed following my evening stretches, I realized that maybe I misinterpreted the abyss. I was looking for answers to come from others over the abyss of the Internet, while others were seeking answers from me. Maybe it was time to participate in the enlightening of the abyss rather than only contributing to its darkness. Renewed energy allowed me to slide back out of bed and move toward my desk. The little red light of my Blackberry was blinking, happily signaling to me that more messages had come from beyond.

I sighed a deep and heavy breath as my hand slid across my phone. Tapping the screen, four more messages appeared, requesting information from me, but nothing from him. Laughing aloud, I decided that it was time to give some people that I cared about some answers that they were no doubt searching for in the abyss. Looking into the black-and-white flashing phone, I saw my reflection. I saw a smile and a sparkle in my eyes as I prepared to send back to those requesting information what perhaps they needed from the abyss. And for me, the abyss would no longer be a place within which I would search for answers.

7 Loss

We have all lost something. For some of us, it is one of our beloved earrings. And in losing it, we are left with only one earring as a painful reminder of what we once owned and enjoyed. But what does the painful reminder mean? Maybe we are fearful that the loss of the earring will also mean the loss of the memory from the joy of the purchase or trying my best to speak Spanish whine I was just learning it in order to purchase the pair. Or maybe we are afraid to lose the memory of the satisfied desire, the memory that preceded the purchase; the walk with a dear friend through the streets of Toledo, stopping at every shop trying to find just the right earrings to capture the joy of the trip. Or perhaps it may mean the loss of the memory of a loved one who gifted the pair to us at just the right moment in our life.

Loss can also be the feeling felt over losing some sort of athletic match that we knew we should and could have won; an interview for a job we felt cheated out of; or simply the painful reminder of a lost childhood as we listen to a child screaming in the park as she watches her balloon float away, far up to meet the clouds.

We all know loss.

Tonight, I think of the loss of those I love. I think of Mark, blown up in Beirut for a reason I still don't understand. I think of my middle school classmate, Cheryl, who jumped off the grain elevator, and I feared it was because I didn't pick her to be on my dodgeball team when I was made captain earlier that day. I think of my high school sweetheart's best friend, who killed himself for an unknown reason. I think of Christopher, Marie, Jason, Lynette, Paul, and Janet; all people who were taken from me, from life, from those who love them much earlier than I think they should have been. I feel the pain of the loss of their life, of their energy, of the joy they brought to the world, of the robbery of their youth.

Then, I think of Leigh Ann, who was raped at nineteen, and Lynette, who was raped at thirty-three, and me, what age was that anyway? It doesn't really matter. I think of the loss of innocence, of security, of trust, of hope, of joy, of dreams.

And then I think of the loss of love. I think of my divorces, my friends' divorces, my girlfriend's split from her lesbian partner of seventeen years, of the "perfect" couples in my life whose unions ended with separation, and of all the weddings of friends; I wonder whether they are really going to "make it."

And then I wonder why we even try at all. Why do we try to pick ourselves up after one type of loss, only to experience another? I think of Cheryl, who discovered her husband's adultery and then returned to her home, which was burned to the ground by an arsonist. She lost twenty-seven years of her married life's memories. She lost all of her material possessions. She lost hope of ever being able to replace all of her possessions. Or did she lose that when she discovered her husband's affair?

We all know loss.

I think of children losing parents and the unthinkable, of parents losing children. I think of lost limbs and lost memory, lost speech and lost sight, lost hearing and lost understanding. I think of the tragedy of loss and the resonating pain of it through every fiber of our being until I can't think or feel any longer.

And then in the midst of the despair of it all, of all the losses of my own and of those whom I love so dearly, I feel a tender persistent voice of encouragement that allows me to simply keep trying. It is a voice that calls to me in the darkest night and the darkest hour, and it simply says, "Choose again."

In those moments, I can dry my tears and look up to the heavens. I can shake off despair and mourning and pain, and I can choose gratitude for having had the person in my life even for just a moment. I can choose gratitude for the lessons that were learned. I can choose peace from the memories that were love inspired, and I can choose compassion and forgiveness in those that were not. I can choose joy, and I can choose to trust another just one more time.

Loss will always be there, as will my ability to choose how I perceive it. So my joy resides in how I choose to perceive loss. I know I have only begun to experience my share of loss; whether I am ready for the next loss that I see coming in my rear view mirror or the one that I don't see as it shatters my windshield. I will experience more loss; it is inevitable. Yet, I get to choose how I experience it after it has occurred.

I can choose to see loss, recognize it in others, embrace it, hold it, be with it, and then let it go, or I can choose to ignore it; even if it is for just a few more months. I can choose how I view loss. I can choose to be transformed by it in a positive way, or I can cave in to the grief of it. I know that I can choose to experience the power of its capability to transform my life, my perspectives of what I need versus what I want. I can make all kinds of stories about what I have lost and revel in those stories that will more than likely cause me more and more pain. Or I can say, "Well, that was a hell of a lesson I just learned. I don't think I need to learn that one anymore," and move forward in love and compassion.

Thus, while I don't embrace loss, I will shun it no more. I won't fear it, nor will I resist it. I will view it as a significant marker on my journey to true abundance. I will be open to its lessons, open to its pain, and more importantly, open to the joys of the lessons learned and won through loss. I will simply ask, what am I learning from this loss? How am I transforming from this loss? How will I love more deeply by having experienced this loss? And I will smile at "loss" as I would smile at a friend who has returned to ask for more favors when I thought I had no more to give. Abundance, when fueled by love, always has more to give. And genuine overflowing gratitude is a way that we can walk in love.

8 Showing Up

"You are absolutely never allowed to date again!" Lelina yelled loudly, interrupting all the conversation in the room. I glanced away from the tray of appetizers I was arranging on the kitchen counter and began to strike my infamous pose: one hand on the hip and the other hand with the finger pointed straight up in the air, when Lelina interrupted my move with another announcement.

"No, Marilee, I am serious. You are never to date again. You suck at it!" With that second announcement, the informal chatter was immediately replaced with a symphony of women's laughter. I surrendered from my full-on attitude pose and resumed tending to the appetizers.

It was girl's night out, and tonight, we were gathered in my home to watch a chick flick; we rented movies but never watched them because we were too engrossed in our conversations with each other to remember we even rented a movie in the first place. My beautiful friends were just arriving, and I was busy setting out trays of appetizers while they were opening bottles of wine.

I had just told the story of my latest dating disaster, in which I had just found out that yet another very nice man I was dating was, in fact, well, married. This was the third time this had happened to me since I had moved to San Diego. As the laughter died down, Krishna chimed in.

"Ya know, Marilee, Lelina may have a point here. Ya gotta wonder how this keeps happening to you."

Krishna barely finished her thought when Briana joined in. "Haven't I taught you anything?" she asked. "You don't ask them if they are married. You wait until they are comfortably settled into conversation with you and then you ask them, 'Is there anyone in your life who would be upset if they walked in and saw you sitting here with me in this way?'"

"Seriously?" Sherrel responded. "You have to ask people you are dating that kind of question these days? I am so glad I am happily married and not in the dating world." Several of my friends' heads nodded in agreement, even the unpartnered ones. I stopped arranging my fine selection of Trader Joe's appetizers for a moment, not to join in the conversation but to write down the question Briana had just shared with me, and I intended not to write it on a notepad but in my Blackberry. *That way,* I thought, *I would always have it with me when I needed it.*

"What are you doing?" Lelina questioned, noticing me typing furiously on my Blackberry.

"I am writing down Briana's question," I responded innocently and sincerely, not even looking up. However, I could feel Lelina's scowl on the back of my neck, and it sent shivers down my spine. I reluctantly turned around, gently setting my Blackberry on the counter and pushing it away from Lelina's scowl as if I thought her gaze could remove the words I had just typed. I peered into her face. I could now see the scowl in full view, and the shivers were still running down my spine. I knew what that scowl meant; we were all about to receive one of Lelina's lessons. Lelina was famous for sharing lessons that were taught in a way that challenged the very core of who you are and who you are becoming.

Lelina must have felt all of our discomfort as her scowl gave way to a smile and she chided me, "Marilee, someone just like you probably existed centuries ago, someone who couldn't date well, and that is what led to the creation of arranged marriages." With that, we all burst into laughter again, and the lively conversations resumed.

Kylie now shared her advice that I should join an on-line dating service instead of resorting to meeting men on airplanes. Several friends shared their successes with this process. However, I explained to them that I had tried that and while I saw the value in participating in on-line dating, it wasn't for me. I really hated the feeling that I was at a buffet table waiting to sample all the delicacies before me. I hated buffets. The selections all seemed appealing and the pressure to choose felt overwhelming. So I ended up sampling too much, and then I ended up overeating. And then, well, then I felt uncomfortable. Seriously, that is what on-line dating felt like to me. All these beautiful souls to meet, the pressure to select just one to date, but you don't, and you overselect, and then you feel uncomfortable. I didn't want to do it.

Maria encouraged me to join one of those dating services, the kind that does the "shopping" for you and then you date whom they select for you. I hated to admit this to my friends, but I had tried that too. They wondered why I didn't like that option. I explained to them that I felt it was too stressful. Again, here were all these beautiful souls who desired to be partnered and had paid to have someone select them for a date, and then you are not interested in them or vice versa. It is hard to feel good about being rejected when you are already way invested in meeting someone and you have all those preconceived expectations. For me, it was a recipe for disaster. Suffice it to say, I didn't like how that felt either. I didn't know how to honor a human being fully, including myself, in this kind of arrangement. So, I just didn't want to do it.

"Let's face it, gang," I announced to the room full of my fabulous friends. "I am screwed. I should do as Lelina says and quit dating."

That announcement brought another roar of laughter, and I realized right then and there that as hopeless of a case as I may truly be, they were never going to give up on me. And they didn't. They teased me for a while longer and then the conversation turned to a topic that only friends who truly love each other can discuss.

"So, how do you think you are showing up, Marilee?" Lelina queried.

"Huh?" I responded as I dropped three of the twelve stuffed mushroom turnovers onto the floor because my spatula was too small to manage the scoop I had attempted.

"How do you think you are showing up?" she continued. "Why is that you are attracting unavailable men into your life?" Wham! The words hit me as if I had taken the spatula itself and slapped it upside my head.

Lelina continued to explain that how we show up in a room allows us to be open to meeting someone, be closed off to a conversation, or send a message we don't want to send. She spoke of one friend who had showed up in a manner where he moved from showing an interest in meeting someone to being obsessed with meeting someone. In doing so, he was no longer showing up with open compassion, but an obsession to just meet someone. Lelina then mentioned another friend who showed up closed; her arms literally crossed in front of her and a posture that was so rigid, giving off judgmental and condescending energy. Other than Buddha and Jesus and perhaps a few other spiritual masters, who can feel welcomed in that kind of space? Of course her friend's beauty and brilliance could not be recognized under such a defensive screen.

Lelina's examples caused me to consider how I show up in my own life. How do I show up as I travel on an airplane? Do I show up flirtatious yet distant, making myself attractive to unavailable men? How do I show up to my students? Do I show up too busy for them to talk to me or too distracted to listen to their concerns? How do I show up to my boss, to those I love, and to those I desire to meet? Am I even conscious of that? Am I intentional about it? Am I showing up in love and joy or in fear and trepidation? And when I realize that the way I desire to show up is not how I am showing up, do I have the courage to look within to find why I may be showing up in this manner? And if I can't figure it out right then, do I have the courage to graciously exit the building until I can find the time for self-reflection?

What a gift this night with my dear girlfriends was to me. What a gift to be able to be so vulnerable and receive such wise counsel and loving support. *How many people have this gift in their lives?* I wondered as I drifted off to sleep that night.

That night, I had a dream. I was feeling broken by the relationship I had just experienced, and I had dreamt that I was a fragile egg. I had fallen and my shell had shattered, splintering into several pieces on the ground. I immediately recognized that my shell was beyond repair. As I lay on the hard unforgiving ground, my tender and vulnerable egg broken and bleeding yolk and egg white, I realized that I was still intact. While my shell had been shattered beyond repair and my yolk was mixed with the white, I was still together.

As I lay on the ground, shattered yet still whole, I heard approaching footsteps and realized that if I didn't pull myself up, I would be stepped on. *Perhaps then, if I were to be stepped on, I would truly be ruined,* I thought to myself within my dream. So, I breathed a deep and lasting breath. And I pulled myself upright. The shell was still lying on the ground as I pulled myself upright. My yolk and white were mixed, and I looked almost transparent. However, I moved forward with an agility I never thought I had. I moved forward with a strength that didn't seem possible for one who appeared so fragile and transparent. As I strode forward on the concrete walkway, not really knowing where I was going, I walked with confidence and I thought to myself, *I wonder how I am showing up now.*

9   The Shifts

It is an interesting thing to think, as we reflect back on our lives, about when we actually made a "shift" or a transition. It usually happens something like this.

Curious Friend: "So when did you begin to realize that your life was all about stupidity and you had no real meaning and you wanted to do something about that?"

Me: "Well, I guess it was when I was lying flat on my back in my bed, not really able to move very well, and my crazy-ass boyfriend was trying to break into my home. It was New Year's Eve, or perhaps New Year's Day in the wee hours of the morning, and he was yelling obscenities at me while pounding on my front door. He was saying that I was the biggest sorry ass loser he ever knew, breaking up with him on New Year's Eve. I was listening to this, frightened to my core, but my disease had me in so much pain and the numbness was so intense that I couldn't even reach the telephone to call 911. I realized I had not turned on the home alarm when I got home earlier that evening, and I was so afraid he would break a window and enter my home, and I would be helpless to defend myself, so I began to pray."

Curious Friend, looking dumb-founded: "Seriously, that really happened to you?"

Me: "Yeah, are you kidding me? You can't make shit like that up. But then, again, I guess the quest to really figure out what was going on in my life happened when I began to wonder how exactly could I appear in the world to be successful yet be so very sad and confused inside; that question really started six months prior to the New Year's Eve incident. You see, my divorce was only a few days from being final when I met this amazing couple in Costa Rica. They could sense my scattered energy and asked me if I had ever had a reading. I had no idea what they were talking about, so I replied, 'Why yes, I read a great deal, thank you. To what reading are you referring?' They, of course, explained to me what an energy reading was, and my curiosity was piqued. I enthusiastically consented to a reading. I was astounded that this couple I had just met knew stuff in my life that I had shared with no one. They saw the history of physical and sexual abuse, they saw the driven desire to please and to achieve, and they saw a very confused, scattered, and very afraid little girl trying her best to 'act' like she had it all together. I came away from that moment aware that there was a world I knew nothing about, and I was curious to learn more about it."

Curious Friend: "So, your shift began prior to the disease that left you bed-ridden; it occurred when you met this couple in Costa Rica?"

Me: "No, the disease never left me bed-ridden; it was just at its height about six months after the Costa Rica trip. I think it is coincidental that six months after the Costa Rica trip was the incident with the crazy-ass boyfriend that I told you about prior. That New Year's Eve had been a long day, and the disease isn't kind to me when I get really tired.

"The time that I really lost total feeling in my legs and a lot of my arms was this past fall, after I had returned from Japan; I was still reeling from my engagement ending. That is when I was taken to the hospital because I couldn't move my legs at all and could barely move my arms."

Curious Friend: "So, was that the shift, then? When you collapsed at the Starbucks and your student had to call 911 using your phone because your arms didn't work and neither did your legs?"

Me: "Oh no, I think the shift that led to that happened ten months prior when I was on Maui and pledged to be my own best partner. You see, I was feeling down in the dumps because Don was supposed to be there with me, but we broke up four months prior and all I could think about on this gorgeous island, on my forty-fifth birthday, was how great it would be if Don or some special guy was with me, but they weren't. So, I decided then and there to choose a different set of thoughts. Thus, I chose right on the beach, on my birthday morning walk before I went to work, that I could be my own best partner; that I didn't need a partner to treat me like a princess on my birthday; I could do it myself. And so I made a pledge to myself to be my best partner. I bought a Maui pearl for myself to seal the commitment to myself and I …"

Curious Friend: "Uh, Marilee, uh, I don't mean to interrupt, but I am trying to find out when you felt that the shift or transition or realization that you needed to awaken your spiritual self occurred. So was there a pivotal moment in time when that happened?"

I heartily laughed, half embarrassed by my ramblings and half just completely amused by the question.

Me: "Sweetie, my head is so thick, there were a thousand moments that were presented to me to awaken to my spiritual self. And a thousand and one times, I acted upon those awakenings, and then I forgot about them and slid back into my ego-led life. Even right now, as we chat, I risk sliding back into an ego-driven life. I just now trust that the awakening lesson, the moment of the shift, will yet come again.

"These awakening moments do, however, seem to be growing in intensity; it's as if God has raised her voice. Yet, I know that that isn't the case. I just keeping asking for a course correction before I get off course, and I am grateful it is provided. I am just so dense, it seems that it just has to come in a pretty traumatic form. So, does that answer your question?"

Curious Friend: "Not really, but thank you for visiting. I am going to go ask Elisa the same question. I think she will give me a clearer answer."

Hugging my gorgeous friend, I giggled to myself as I saw her stroll toward Elisa and ask her the same question.

I watched the interaction from a distance. Elisa tossed her long flowing curls as her head rolled back, laughing aloud at the question posited. *Yup,* I thought to myself. *She will give a clearer answer.*

Awakenings, shifts, transition opportunities are all around us all the time. We respond and then we quickly forget about them as we slide back into our sleep. If we remember to invite another awakening, it will come. And perhaps we can share our awakenings with our friends and ask them to remind us when we act as if we have forgotten. Wouldn't that be the essence of living an accountable life, to share such things with those who can remind us to walk the path we believe we are meant to walk? As I write this, I am inviting another awakening, yet inviting it without all the drama of the former ones. Furthermore, I am sharing these lessons with those I trust to remind me when I stray from my path. I invite the awakenings, and I trust they will come in the moments when I slide back into the sneaky tricks of my ego-driven life.

10 Discovering Relationship

"If you do end up having only a year to live, I will have sex with you, but you have to provide a doctor's note proving you're about to die."

"Are you fucking kidding me?" I responded over my cell phone to Dan, my former lover and now very dear friend. "Are you serious? If I am dying of ovarian cancer and I only have a year to live, I have to provide you with a doctor's note in order to have sex with you?"

"Absolutely," he responded, his voice showing no emotion, "and it better be official. I am a captain, ya know, I can verify these things."

With that, we both burst into laughter.

The Captain—Captain Dan—and I had just arrived at our separate homes, me after him, following our earlier dinner together at some hole-in-the wall pasta shop we had never noticed before. We had met our friend Laura prior to dinner for some hot yoga that totally kicked my butt, and afterward, we decided that in order to recover before driving home, we had to find a glass of wine and some carbs and protein. We wound up at a pasta place across from the yoga studio, a place none of us had ever even seen before

At dinner, we talked to our much younger friend, Laura, about the latest adventure in her dating relationship with her boyfriend. She shared about the stage they were in in their dating relationship and questions that she had. Dan and I, of course, offered her wine-induced advice that, while questionable, basically revolved around simply being true to herself. As I sat back and watched two of my priceless friends exchange conversation, I thought, *Wow, it really is that simple. Just be honest with yourself and then be honest with him. If you don't know where you are, then just simply state that. If you don't know what you want, then simply state that. And for heaven's sake, don't do anything that you think you should do like have sex with him, just because he wants it; figure out how you feel about it first and then talk about it.*

The conversation then transitioned to Dan's recent break-up with his high school heartthrob. I was so sad about this news. Even though I had that *Oh, I wish that were me* boulder in the pit of my stomach when I first saw them together, I had grown to really love seeing Dan and Allison together. I could see their connection, and I loved how happy he looked when they were dancing or simply walking into a room. The joy on his face and on hers had brought joy to my heart. So, in this moment, I was genuinely and deeply saddened to learn that they had decided to split up.

As I listened to Dan talk about the transition in their relationship, I couldn't help feel preoccupied with my own thoughts. It was, after all, only four days after I learned that I needed to have my left ovary removed. The blob that the doctor and I thought would go away had grown two centimeters in two months and darkened in color; it was not a good sign. While I had done my own research on ovarian cancer and realized that I had all the symptoms, I was recalling the doctor's positive outlook that would occur after surgery; I couldn't help think that I may not have many more opportunities to do hot yoga with these two and then subsequently share love stories with them over pasta dishes and cheap wine.

At that moment, I heard Dan share with Laura the story of the Buddhist monk who experienced bad things and good things all the while not deciding whether they were bad or good, even though the people around him determined them to be thus. I giggled aloud as I heard Dan's version dramatically differ from the story I had read, and I then realized that this is probably how all the stories of Jesus had gotten fucked up. They got messed up in translation. They were probably told and retold while people were drinking wine after a long day of work.

The giggles resulting from my own private thoughts did not interrupt this pair's conversation, so I returned to my own thoughts. Dan's story was timely for me. *In a few weeks*, I thought, *I am having my left ovary removed and most likely the rest of the female reproductive system, where three blobs are finding a healthy growing venue. Yet, today is the first day in over a week that I have been able to keep down my food. Is this good news after bad news or is it simply the way it is?*

"It is all about who you are in relationship to it," I heard Dan say as I came back to the table from my thoughts.

Yes, I thought. *It is. Who am I in relationship to the tumors in my ovary? Who am I in relationship to being able to keep down my food today? Who am I in relationship to the pain that courses across my abdomen and my back? Who am I in relationship to my fatigue? Who am I in relationship to these gorgeous friends sitting across from me? Who am I in relationship to the food and wine that rests in front of me? Who am I in relationship to the homeless person who just now walked past the window?*

As I sat up to rejoin the conversation, the delightful and very patient manager approached our booth to let us know that her staff really had to go home, and therefore, she really needed us to leave. We smiled graciously, irresponsibly gulped down our remaining wine (because we all believe it is a mortal sin to waste it and at this point in my life, I ain't taking any chances with sin), and left the charming hole-in-the-wall establishment.

As we crossed the street and strolled back to our cars, Laura and Dan still fully engaged in their conversation, I paused and looked back toward the pasta place and wondered how I had never seen it before. Then I smiled and wondered if it would be there the next time I returned to this yoga studio or whether it was a mystical place just created for tonight so that we could have the conversation that was just meant for us to have.

I don't know, I smiled to myself, *but it is neither good nor bad, it just is. And who am I in relationship to it? Perhaps a woman that has a year to live or perhaps a woman who will be taking Laura's kids there on a random Saturday afternoon fifteen years from now.*

"Dan," I giggled, managing to pull myself together over the hilarious realization that I would have to provide a doctor's note in order to have sex with him should I die in a year, "I love you."

"I love you too, kiddo. Get some rest and keep your food down," he responded lovingly.

I giggled some more, ready to start a new thread of conversation with him that addressed the reason why he may feel he needed a doctor's note so that I wouldn't throw up on him while we were having sex in the last year of my life, but I refrained. Instead, I smiled, wished him well, and clicked the button on my cell phone to end the call.

Who am I in relationship to sex? I now thought. *I often confuse sex for a need to be intimate with my God.* After a long pause, I decided to take hot sex off my bucket list. I am so richly blessed by beautiful friends, friends whose company reminds me of how intimate I am with God.

I have a whole lot of love in my life. *I think the question really is, who am I in relationship to love?* One year left, five, or twenty-five. *I am love in relationship to love.* Neither good nor bad, just is.

11 Fire Yoga

"Yes, let's go to yoga tonight before we go out ... brilliant idea," I said enthusiastically over the phone to Linda as I continued to check my e-mail at my desk. "What time works best for you?" I politely asked and then wondered why I did. As usual, I was so tightly scheduled that I wasn't actually sure at ten o'clock in the morning, the time we were talking on the phone, just when I would eat my meals that day, let alone pee. Thus, I only had about an hour to fit in a yoga class before we connected with our friends later that evening to celebrate our January birthdays.

I didn't really listen to Linda's response to my question, where she was telling me when she was available, because just after realizing that I really only had one hour for yoga that day, I became further distracted by an e-mail from a colleague. My colleague was letting me know that even though there were three weeks for her to print out eighteen dissertation research posters for our doctoral students' research symposium, she really didn't have time, and so she was letting me know that she couldn't do it, via e-mail.

"Unfucking believable!" I yelled into the phone, forgetting I was on the phone with Linda because I was preoccupied with the e-mail. Linda, obviously and understandably, had no clue what I was talking about; she stopped her conversation abruptly. It was, unfortunately, in that moment that she stopped her conversation that I realized that I had not been listening to her. Well, now I was aware of that, and so was she. An awkward silence followed.

"Uh, Linda?" I inquired. "Are you still there?" More awkward silence. "Linda? I am sorry, what were you saying?"

"Geezuz, Marilee, how can you profess to be a yogi and be such a bitch?" Linda asked with great calm. That question actually made me laugh as it brought back an image of a bumper sticker I had seen earlier that week. The bumper sticker had read, "You call me a bitch like it's an insult." I had wondered how hilarious it would be to place that bumper sticker on the back of my Jeep, right next to the "Namaste" sticker.

Linda was not amused by my laughter, so I spent the next fifteen minutes apologizing to her, explaining that my exclamation was not directed at her and her schedule. It was a reaction to an e-mail I was reading when I should have been listening to her. My nonpresence with Linda not only did not honor her being, it demonstrated that I was so not living out my morning prayer, which invited a reminder that how I treat others is how I treat myself. Or had the prayer been in effect after all?

After further apologizing to Linda, we selected a later yoga time than what she suggested so I wouldn't have to rush to get there. Linda further offered to text our friends to let them know we would be later in meeting them, because we were going to a later yoga class. We just didn't want to have to rush anywhere that evening.

I hung up the phone, literally singing praises for Linda and the beauty that she consistently resonated. She was living the being that I so desired to emulate. A reminder popped up on my monitor, which I had been ignoring the last fifteen minutes so I could focus on Linda's voice; I was already late to my next meeting. So I rushed off.

Later that evening, I walked into the yoga studio, saw Linda standing in the check-in line, and embraced her with a warm and loving hug. We were getting ready to check into our one-hour heated level 2 Vinyassa yoga class, and we were chatting excitedly about our busy day, about how glad we were that we had made time for yoga, and how much we really needed it after the week we had experienced. And then we chatted about the difference it made in not having to rush to get there. We further commented about how fun it would be to meet our friends later, at one of our favorite wine bars, for a celebration of life. All was going smoothly until we got to the counter.

"Checking in for the ninety-minute hot yoga class or the yoga sculpt class?" the gorgeous young female yoga teacher asked, with all the effervescent and genuine charm that ever existed on the face of the planet.

"Huh?" I responded with such flat affect that I even bored myself with my own response.

"Well, if you want the yoga sculpt class, you have six minutes to get changed and into the classroom, so I think you better go to the hot yoga class instead," she said, her jet black hair bouncing along with each bright word.

"Huh?" was the best I could come up with.

Fortunately Linda intervened, saying, "We'll go to the hot yoga class." She said it with great confidence, yet I was not fooled. I noticed her glance at me as she spoke. It was the glance that mirrored exactly what I was thinking. Hot yoga? Ninety minutes of 105 degree temperature? We would be lucky to come out of there alive.

Is she nuts? I thought to myself. I am going to die in there. And I am going to die prior to having my birthday celebration glass of wine. This sucks.

"Excuse me," I interrupted Linda and asked the fit and slender instructor as politely as I could for someone who was panicking to save her own life. "Uh, I know you are busy," I began politely. "And I know this line behind me is growing with each 'huh' I utter, but what happened to the C2 power Vinyassa, non-105 degree temperature class that is typically offered at this time?"

"We recently changed our schedule in response to the member survey we sent out in December," she smiled as gloriously as she had greeted us. With that, I was distracted from my need to survive by three thoughts. *One, how was it that every yoga instructor I had ever met in this studio was drop dead gorgeous? Two, I love that they did a survey; I wonder who designed it and I wonder if in the future, I can barter yoga classes in exchange for assisting them with survey design and analysis. And three, was death by yoga the universe's reward for my not rushing to yoga?*

As we completed our check-in and sauntered toward the shower room, I knew Linda and I were thinking the exact same thing. We could so easily ditch out of here, out the side exit door, and head to the wine bar. Or we could risk our well-being and actually do this class. She and I didn't need to speak a word as we glanced away from the exit door and looked at each other. I felt like I was on my death march. There were moments of fleeing in both of our eyes and moments of thinking that we might be entering our last great adventure. We decided to go for it; we decided to go to class.

As we entered the yoga classroom, where silence was sacred and signs hung all around the studio as reminders that silence was the norm, I began to giggle. I couldn't help it. I was entering a ninety-minute hot yoga (105 degrees as a reminder) classroom. I hadn't attempted hot yoga since I had collapsed only four months earlier, but that thought was quickly dismissed by another. I had had lentils for my very late lunch. So now, instead of trying not to fart for sixty minutes, I was going to have to hold it in for ninety minutes. In addition, after the week I had had, I was really looking forward to hanging with my friends and celebrating life, sharing the lessons we had learned, and receiving encouragement. That was now delayed even longer. So all I could do, well, was giggle.

Fortunately (or unfortunately), Linda and I found a place next to each other near the door. Linda giggled as well as she leaned over and said, "At least we are next to the escape route."

That comment turned my giggle into a laugh, and yogis were beginning to glance our way as if to signal that we were breaking the silence vow and it was not appreciated. That made us giggle even more, as we decided that tonight, our role was to give everyone in the room an opportunity to practice their nonreaction. Our joy did not last long, however. As the class began to fill, we had to scoot away from the door to make room for those entering late. I couldn't help but think that these were people who were rushing to yoga and benefiting now by their tardiness with easy escape access to the door and easy access to cooler air. *Was this another funny joke that the universe was playing?*

My mind was so not in the best place when class began. I just couldn't clear my mind; it was loud with chatter, and the chatter grew into a roar as the room increased in heat. I was "doing" yoga but I wasn't. Instead, I noticed those yogis who were wearing stylish outfits and those who weren't. I wondered how my Costco yoga outfit would stand up to both sets of folks on a scale of one to ten by the fashion police. And then I noticed that the outfits all looked the same, as we began to sweat in them. I noticed all the guys in the classroom and wondered which were single and straight and which were not. I examined people's asanas and determined which ones I would adjust if I were teaching the class and admired those who needed no adjustment. I wondered how many yogis were young enough to be my kids and wondered if I was the oldest person in the room. My mind was all over the place.

Good thing I went to the bathroom just before class. I wonder if I will need to go before class ends. Is that a cramp I feel? Okay, breathe into it. Oh my, there is another one. Okay, breathe into it. I so should not have eaten those lentils. I hope we don't do an inversion. Is that a pain in my chest or is this asana just creating more pressure there? Am I having a heart attack or did I just forget to breathe? Hey, is that one of my students or am I starting to hallucinate? Ha, I am still going and the gal who is half my age in front of me is in child's pose. I so rock. Wait a minute, yoga is not about comparison. Quit comparing yourself to others. Focus. Wow, look at her flexibility. She so rocks. Where did Linda go? Did she leave the room? Hey, what is going on with my stomach? I think I am starting to feel sick.

As I became convinced that I was a lost cause for this class, I heard the instructor's commanding voice say, "And what are you choosing now? Are you choosing to listen to your ego?" I began to wonder whether a sense of humor was a part of ego or a part of spirit. After all, I was laughing at my failure in class. The yoga continued, and I heard her announce again, "What are you choosing now? What are you choosing in this moment?" *In this moment,* I thought, *I am choosing not to throw up my lentils!*

More hot yoga, and I wondered whether I would make it. I wondered whether anyone had ever died in a hot yoga class. She asked again, "What are you choosing now? What are you choosing in this moment?"

In this moment, I thought, *I am choosing survival.* But then the laughter in my head that came from this mental response created a space for a different answer. *I am choosing to be here, even if by accident,* I thought. The voice continued, *And if I believe there are no coincidences, then I have chosen to be here.* That thinking created new space for a different thought. *I choose to be here.* The yoga practice suddenly became much lighter, and the room became much less hot.

Now, I was finally engaged in my yoga practice. I had no idea how much time it had taken me to get there, but perhaps I needed that ninety-minute class for just this reason; for the reason that on that day, I would need more time to get out of my head. There are no mistakes, and there are no coincidences.

And then the instructor asked, "What are you choosing now? What are you choosing in this moment? Are you choosing yes? Are you choosing transformation?" I had finally engaged in my yoga practice. I was not going to die today in this 105 degree room. So now, when she asked that question, rather than my smart-ass earlier replies, I now wanted to scream out a joyful "Yes!" I wanted to exclaim to her that I chose yes to transformation, and as Baron Baptiste suggests, I chose yes when I wondered how I was going to get through something. All I really have to do in every difficult asana, in every difficult moment, all I have to do is choose yes.

12 Greater Good

"It's all for the what?" Mike said as his fixed gaze stared down at his size 13 feet sliding along the pavement, kicking up sand purposefully whenever possible. I looked over to study his face, determining whether he really wanted me to go on or had grown tired of my rambling. As I studied him, I couldn't help notice how much taller my cousin was compared to me. I mean, he stands over six feet tall; he is tall, period. My cousin Mike and I consistently joked about the possibilities that contributed to our extended family only having two members who reached over five feet, nine inches, and he turned out to be the taller of those two. My lengthy pause caused him to cut short his shuffle and look up at me.

"What? Seriously, what? Come on, pretend I am a simple man, pretend I am Bohemian and slow, and well, just explain it to me one more time, will you?"

I laughed aloud as I chided him that no pretending was needed.

"You are a dumb male Bohunk, Cuz. I don't need to pretend." With that, he threw his long arm around me and pulled me into him for a warm, loving hug that only Mike was capable of giving. He knew I was joking. He knew how much I thought of his gifts, and that embrace communicated to me all I needed to know to be sure that he knew I was teasing him.

"Okay, I'll give it to you one more time, but we'll need to sit down so I can have your full attention instead of your drifting gazes toward the babes on the beach." With that, we strolled up onto an old wooden deck that faced the ocean. The deck belonged to a Pacific Beach joint, it was a well-worn deck and a well-known location. As we settled into our bar stools that overlooked the splintered deck railing facing the ocean, I wasn't so sure this was the best spot to have such a serious conversation, but I could tell by the emotion on Mike's face, it was absolutely the time.

After ordering our adult beverages from the very attractive waitress—who I noticed because Mike repeatedly pointed her attractiveness out to me—I began.

"Okay, I think this all might make a little more sense if I give it a little context." He nodded approvingly, and I proceeded to take him back two nights ago to a Friday when he, a bunch of friends, and I had been out dancing at one of our favorite San Diego nightclubs.

I asked him if he noticed that night how each one of our friends were invited to dance. Mike, smiling slightly at the memories from the evening, gave me another approving nod, encouraging me to go on without his interrupting. I proceeded to explain how Kim, our friend who is in a committed long-distance relationship, practically jumped into the arms of anyone who would ask her. She was ready to have a blast, and that made her the most popular dancer of the night, something we became a little concerned about as the evening wore on and men's interest in her intensified.

Samantha, on the other hand, was guarded, so guarded that when I was on the dance floor looking back at her bar stool perch, I could have sworn she was surrounded by a nine-foot picket fence with barbed wire at the top. And Idina, dressed to kill and looking rather inviting, appeared to shrivel in utter terror when even the nicest looking guy invited her onto the dance floor. At one point when I looked back at Idina, I thought she had been physically assaulted. However, after further study, I realized that her behavior had only been a response to an invitation to dance from the cleanest-cut looking man I had ever seen walk into that club; his invitation just freaked her out. In a matter of minutes, the way each one of our three beloved friends received another into their life, even the momentary life of an invitation to a four-minute public dance, was intended to mark the manner in which they would remember their entire evening experience and, perhaps worse, fold into their already inaccurate perceptions of who they really are.

Mike turned his bar stool away from the gorgeous view of the ocean and began to recite his shared observations and subsequently what he did to ease each one of them into a more centered way of being.

"Exactly!" I shouted as he finished his story of how he helped each friend feel more comfortable in their own space, more centered, and more at peace in their own skins. My enthusiastic affirmation almost sent him tumbling backward in his stool. He caught his balance, as he always does, and leaned forward, inviting an explanation with only his gaze.

"That is what I have been trying to tell you, me dear Cuzin. You are a pillar of centeredness with an amazing ability for outreach. As such, you see people struggling to gain the ability to be comfortable in their own skin. And you, my dear friend, have the gift to help them find that comfort. You coach them into bringing forward their own beauty, and you provide them with an environment where they feel safe to let it shine. And you do this all in a matter of minutes."

He nodded quietly in humble agreement, so I continued.

"The challenge, my priceless cousin, is that when you show up in this way for folks, some of them mistake your facilitating their own ability to be beautiful and comfortable in their own skin as something that only you can do for them. Thus, their expectations and demands for your attention and time increase, causing you stress and a feeling that you have just done something wrong instead of something wondrous."

"Yes," he blurted out, now causing me to sit back on my stool, almost tumbling right onto my drunk neighbor. "Yes, that is how I feel. Oh my God, yes; that is exactly how I feel."

We paused our conversation long enough to gaze toward the ocean—only to spot some middle-aged, overweight, very white guy strip down to the full Monty as he changed out of his swimming trunks and into his shorts. We looked away in horror, and then we looked at each other and burst out laughing.

"I really did not need to see that," Mike mumbled.

I couldn't respond. I was laughing so hard, I was fully focused now on trying to keep my margarita from shooting out my nose.

When we felt we had somewhat recovered from our unpleasant diversion, we returned to our conversation. Mike explained that he could really see the beauty in folks, and he could also see where they struggled to get in touch with their own gifts. It was natural to him to be able to see others' abilities and coach them into a place where they could shine. It felt good to him to be able to facilitate people coming into a place where they felt comfortable in their own skin. I listened to Mike process what he had just heard, and I was very pleased that he recognized his gifts. Yet, I could sense a discomfort in his voice as he, most likely for the first time, articulated the power of his abilities.

His next sentence sent chills down my spine. "It is an awesome responsibility and a very powerful place for me to be with this gift, isn't it?" he inquired.

I looked down into my watery margarita and then out to the ocean. The sky was so blue and clear, I could see for miles. I saw the clarity in the air and in the water, yet I did not have clarity of thought. I couldn't look at Mike yet; I couldn't respond. I closed my eyes, praying for just the right words. And they arrived. I smiled as I looked toward his still quite inquisitive face.

"There is nothing to be afraid of; just ask the Holy Spirit for guidance to use your gift, to use it all for the greater good."

He grinned from ear to ear. We had come back to the conversation that led us to this very spot on the deck. We sat in silence for a long moment, and then, fearing we may see some other overweight white guy full Monty daylight show, we scurried off the deck and walked back to the Jeep in silence.

As I looked down at Mike's size 13 feet, shuffling on the pavement, kicking up the sand, I knew that he understood his gifts, that he understood that he could continue to facilitate others in finding their own magic, in becoming comfortable in their own skin, and that he would no longer feel responsible to stay beside them as a result. He was free to walk onto the next one, the next being, coaching that person into her own gifts, her own place of beauty. And all this would be done for the greater good.

13 Becoming Unengaged

This vignette is dedicated to the beautiful soul who knocked me off my feet, coming and going.

I met him on the dance floor. Yes, on the dance floor. I literally dragged myself away from work one Friday night, suit and all, to head to a celebration of my dear friend, Idina, who had just finished her doctoral degree. While I was genuinely thrilled for Idina, I was incredibly tired. Just one hour prior to the celebration, I had gone to visit my chiropractor/energy work dude. Whatever magic he was doing that day worked, and I had experienced a huge relief. The huge relief came in the form of tears; I bawled my eyes out. The miracle he performed while I was on his table released within me a powerful sense that I was alone, that I was separate, and that I was unsafe. That feeling led to a thousand tears being shed, and a genuine sense of relief and calm came back to my body. It was magic, yet the crying experience left me feeling exhausted.

That is what I experienced just before Idina's formal academic ceremony. I didn't want to miss it, so I dried my tears, put on some face powder in an attempt to cover all the red (I look like a checkered tablecloth after I cry so deeply), straightened my suit coat, and jumped in my Jeep to drive to the ceremony. I was as present as I could be at the academic ceremony, and Idina looked smashing in her light blue cocktail dress.

At the end of the ceremony, all I wanted to do was go home, crawl into bed, and sleep. But that was not going to happen. Instead, I decided that regardless of how tired I felt, Idina must celebrate in a manner that was worthy of this accomplishment. And since I hadn't been able to plan a proper party, I decided to text all of our friends to have them meet us at our favorite dance hangout. They all dropped what they were doing (except for Tony, who was already at the club, celebrating his high school reunion) and promised to arrive at the appointed time.

It took Idina and me longer to get through the crowds and out of the ceremony, so in order to get to the dance place at the appointed time, we ditched our original dinner plans and settled on the closest Mexican drive-through for a carne asada burrito. It was a hilarious sight, Ildina, in her light blue cocktail dress and me in my navy blue pantsuit, splitting a carne asada burrito and trying to keep the sauce from dripping all over us. I failed miserably.

We arrived at our favorite dance place after the planned time to find it completely packed. There was no place to congregate in celebration of Idina. Just as I began to beat myself up for not having thought this all through better, Tony rescued us. He had cleared a couple of tables among his reunion gathering and invited us to join his celebration. The gang was all there, Idina was thrilled, and it could not have been a more fitting celebration of her accomplishment. Tony's friends joined in fully; it was beautiful. My peace returned, but my energy did not.

Grabbing a seat for myself, I simply enjoyed watching everyone dance and have a good time. I still couldn't get up there to join them; the release had taken everything out of me. However, after much coaxing, I took off my suit coat, grabbed a napkin to wipe the dried salsa off my suit pants, and slowly rose to join my friends on the dance floor, where group dancing is more normal than couples dancing (you gotta love that).

I had just gotten into my groove when I looked up and saw him. Dancing just a few feet away from me was a form of energy that knocked me off my feet; I literally tripped and began to fall. I didn't fall completely; Sarina caught me. His name was Garrison, he was a friend of Tony's who had come back for the high school reunion. The first sight of him almost knocked me off my feet.

I didn't fall completely, not that night; but I did one week later when we met again, this time intentionally; I fell for him intentionally; I fell for Garrison fully on that night.

Garrison had also been married twice before. He was five years my senior and very successful in his work. He was what my friend Pamela would describe as "love on two feet." I had announced to everyone that I was dating Buddha, yet a Buddha that enjoyed both wine and beer.

Garrison laughed heartedly, thought deeply, loved greatly, and gave me the impression that there was nothing, absolutely nothing, that I could ever do that would dissuade him from loving me. He was fit, energetic, handsome, and sexy. He was intelligent, witty, and thoughtful, and he had a delightful sense of humor.

I was never without flowers and never in need of anything with Garrison. He read my books, attended my lectures, and even carried my suitcase when he could accompany me on my business trips. He was not perfect; I knew that, yet he was a manifestation of love like I had never seen before.

That night, one week after we met, he made a ring out of a dollar bill and placed it on my left ring finger. I thought it was sweet; I didn't realize I had just been proposed to.

One month later, he was the only man I wanted to be with, and he began to talk about marriage. Yes, he used the "m" word, the word that had been forbidden from my vocabulary since my second divorce. The "third time is a charm" thing was not something I was willing to try, not in this arena. I didn't believe that marriage would ever be for me, ever.

I was a hypocrite. I could encourage my friends to get back on the horse; I signed up for seminars on "calling in the one" and wrote intention letters on what the one would look like and told myself I would go for it should I meet him. And here I was dating him, but I couldn't speak the "m" word. I couldn't even write it out. I kept asking him, "Are we going to have the 'm' talk again, can't we just do a commitment ceremony instead?" He wanted to get married; it was important to him.

After several conversations with friends serving as mediators, he asked me again, this time via a Skype text, as he was in China and I had just landed in San Diego. Yes, he had proposed to me via text messaging, and this time, I had accepted.

After I typed "Yes" on my Blackberry, a relief and excitement surged through my every cell. I no longer was held hostage by fear of the "m" word. I could say, "Yes, I would be honored to marry you." And I could really feel that I meant it. I was no longer a hypocrite. After knowing each other for only three months, we set the wedding date for one year later at a gorgeous resort in San Diego. I was on cloud nine. I had overcome my fear, and I was looking at my dream straight in the eyes.

One month after our humongous and very public engagement party, the dream died.

Do you remember when you were a kid, and you were swinging on a swing? It was so overwhelmingly joyous to be flying so high up in the sky, carefree, wind blowing in your hair, laughing your heart out, and thinking that life just couldn't get any better. But then you think it would be really fun to jump out of the swing at its highest, so you do.

You are still having a ball, flying through the air, until you land. When you land, you realize that your legs are not underneath you, you are on your belly, face down, mouth full of dirt, eyes tearing up so much you can't see, and then you realize you have a serious pain in your chest. You start to panic, because you can't breathe. Try as hard as you may, you can't get your breath back, you can't even move. You feel completely alone and in pain, but before you even realize it, your friends come over and pick you up, dust you off, and hold you up, feet dangling in midair; your friends literally hold you up and hold on to you, coaching you not to panic but to breathe. You hear distant voices asking you how you are, and then they become clearer. Slowly, ever so slowly, you begin to see again, hear again, and breathe again. You carefully find your feet, stand up, and realize that your friends are still hanging on. You assure them that you are okay, and you are grateful that they are still hanging onto you, holding you up, until they actually see with their own eyes that you can walk on your own.

That is how I felt one week after Garrison let me know that he no longer wanted to marry me. We were driving his belongings down from the great state of Washington to San Diego. We had packed him up, and he was moving in; the wedding was eleven months away. We were laughing, singing, and planning details of our life together, tooling down the road. When we hit the California border, I sensed stress rising in him. I put on my inquiry cap and went about trying to understand what was bothering him.

The only thing left on the list was the wedding. So, for some strange, very weird reason, I asked him if he still wanted to marry me. I have no idea why I asked it, but I did ask it staring down at the one carat princess cut on my left hand.

His response was an announcement that he no longer wanted to marry me. I was too shocked to speak. I didn't see it coming, and I had no idea what had precipitated it. In that moment, I shut down completely; the fortress I had spent five years tearing down had been rebuilt. In an instant, I chose to undo all the progress I had made.

One week after that moment, because of the love of my friends and family, I feel like I have found my breath, can see through the tears, and that the voices of my dear friends are becoming clearer. I still feel and appreciate my dear friends holding me up, and I am grateful.

As I move into this next week, I am reminding myself that I am still Marilee, that my life was good before I met Garrison. It was full of all of my beautiful friends and family, it was filled with love, joy, and beauty. My life was good, and my life will return to good. I can choose that, and I do. The weird part is that, after having met Garrison and experiencing life with him, I feel that I went from living a great movie in black and white to living a great movie in Technicolor/ Blueray/3-D/whatever. I am finding it hard to just be okay with black and white after having lived in Technicolor. The good thing is that now, I get what all the fuss is all about when people talk about love and marriage; cool stuff, powerful stuff. I believe in love now, maybe even more so. Crazy-ass crazy and true.

I still struggle with not really knowing why Garrison changed his mind. Even though we have talked, I don't understand what happened. I think he just got scared, but I don't know. His announcement, which I didn't see coming, scared me. And then my fear-filled response further scared him. On Saturday, Garrison let me know that he was again willing to marry me but I couldn't get past the first change of mind, because I didn't know why that happened. Apparently both love and fear have brought us both to a place where we are no longer comfortable to marry. Yet, we are comfortable transitioning to friendship.

Some of my friends are calling this a tragedy. They feel we are failing each other. They are questioning that if Love is all you need, why can't you just forgive each other and go back to being together? I don't know, I answer. I believe that Love is all you need, and I believe that Love is allowing us to look at each other honestly and say we better not get married. We have more work to do. I just don't see it as a tragedy. Sure, his decision shocked the hell out of me, and my fearful reaction to it shocked the hell out of him and me, and then his fearful reaction to that, well, you get the picture. I am still recovering from the shock of the announcement and the frustration of not understanding why that all happened. I did not see this coming, and therefore, I do not trust what else may be coming in this relationship. That may be a fear-based decision, or it may be wisdom. I honestly don't know. Regardless, confusion is no place from which to enter into a long-term commitment.

There is no tragedy here. Everyone is still alive, and I am learning more about the great complexities that reside in love and fear; in trying to overcome past heartaches to move forward in confidence and in faith; in balancing reason with trust, in responding with intuition rather than memory, and in balancing observation with heartfelt truth. This is a humbling place to stand, and it is a learning opportunity for which I am grateful.

I am so grateful to my dear friends and family for picking me up when I couldn't breathe, for staying by me as I become more confident in my ability to breathe. I am truly grateful.

14 Dream Awakening

I had dinner with Garrison last night at my favorite Italian restaurant, which is within walking distance from my home. Why? Because he had indicated that he wanted to see me and let me know that he was sure I didn't want to see him. He also let me know that he was convinced I wouldn't invest in our friendship after he changed his mind about wanting to marry me. I wanted to prove him wrong in these assumptions, so I agreed to meet with him; besides, I really needed to give him back the engagement ring. I wanted to let go of the pain that looking at it brought.

The dinner felt like a disaster; it was only this morning that I realized it wasn't. He freely shared with me how he was doing when I asked him. I was sincerely at peace to learn that he had a place to put all his furniture that was going to go in my home (the blessing of coming from a family of twelve), he was happy with the spot he had found for his RV (where he lived part of the time just last winter), he was at peace with how the kids were doing, his original home remodels were going as scheduled, and he was enjoying being back to his daily routine that he so cherished this past winter. The only thing that was causing him heartache was watching his beloved sister, Danielle, continue to fail in her fight against cancer. He shared the pain he was experiencing there in detail. I felt his pain deeply, and I know it is incredibly difficult to watch someone you love lose a battle with a horrible disease. I didn't know how to soothe him. I didn't know if there was a correlation with what he was seeing and feeling for Danielle and his decision to call off the wedding, for we had selected Danielle's birthday as our wedding date. I didn't know anything.

Lost and feeling unempowered by my state of not knowing, the conversation abruptly turned toward us. He let me know that his family was disappointed that it didn't work out between us. I didn't ask him what he had told his family, even though I wanted to know; my ego wanted to know how he was describing all that was happening and that had happened, and I had to tell my screaming ego that it was none of her business, that it didn't matter. He wanted to know what my family and friends were saying. He wanted to know if he could reach out to my friends and family and make sure they understood from his perspective that he wanted to get back together and that I was the one keeping it from happening. I reassured him that I communicated the message he had asked me to and that everyone loved him and wished him well. I assured him that the gang of friends was ready to welcome him back in whenever he was ready.

I told him that I really needed to stay away from the conversation of "us"; I was happy to listen more to how he was doing and all, but I wasn't ready to talk about "us." So, he let me know that he didn't have anything more to say. So, I watched him eat his meal in silence. I could no longer eat. I wasn't doing well. The screaming ego was overshadowing my thoughts and my spirit, and I couldn't keep back my tears. The only choice I felt I had was to apologize to him and excuse myself from the dinner table. I left him money for the meal, slid my engagement ring across the table, and told him I just couldn't keep it together any longer. As I got up from the table, he wanted to know if I wanted the roses that he had brought for me and if he could come by my home after he finished his meal. I told him no (I think I might have actually yelled it out as the entire restaurant was looking my way) and left in a rush.

No clarity came last night as I cried myself to sleep. I knew I was not a victim but I had no idea what I was supposed to be learning from all of this. Or, as my friend Cathy asked, "What truth was this drama keeping me from discovering; from what was this drama distracting me?" (I love that question.)

The next morning, I awoke with a heart so heavy that I could barely breathe. *Damn, I thought I was back on my feet, and now I feel like I am eating dirt again.*

I reached for my daily meditation quotes, and this is what I read: "Light and joy and peace abide in you and in all beings. Your sinlessness is guaranteed by God. Connect your self to your Self."[3]

Yeah, right, I thought to myself. *Connect my ego to my spirit; the two don't get along very well right now. So that just ain't going to happen today.*

I prepared to go to yoga, but when I got on the interstate, the traffic was crawling (drizzle in San Diego brings everything to a screeching halt). I knew I wouldn't make it in time for class. Concerned about the emotional state that I was in and that I might try to yell at someone who was undeserving, I pulled off the interstate and drove to Cowles Mountain to go hiking instead. After all, it was only drizzling outside, and that was nothing compared to the storm I was feeling inside my mind.

As I bowed to the mountain in respect of all its life and beauty before beginning my ascent, I prayed that I would understand the meaning of the words, "Light and joy and peace abide in you and all beings. Your sinlessness is guaranteed by God. Connect your self to your Self." The entire way up the mountain, I argued with my head and my heart. Peace seemed the most distant reality, as did any remnant of joy. As I neared the summit, I saw three doves, and then I realized there were four, *no wait, there were seven doves.* I stopped, mouth dropping in shock, joy washing over me. *Seven doves. How cool is that? And look! What is that? A quail. Wait, three quails. Way cool.* More joy swept over me, and I actually smiled.

Reaching the summit, I offered a brief prayer of gratitude for the cleansing rain that was falling on my head, for the birds that I got to see (seven and three), and for the ability, the energy, and the strength to get out of bed and hike. As I descended, it came; the clarity stopped me in my tracks.

Light, joy, and peace abided in me and in all beings. I needed to connect the "self" who feels pain, guilt, heartache, and who feels the need to be right, the need to be angry, the need to not trust; I needed to connect that with the "Self" who is light, joy, peace, and love. But how?

---

3   A Course in Miracles, Lesson 93.

Baron Baptiste's words from a retreat a few weeks earlier came ringing to my ears: "The answer to how is yes."[4]

So I just yelled out a big "Yes!" And I felt … nothing. I laughed aloud at myself and walked on.

As I walked on, mumbling my new mantra, I saw Garrison across from me at the dinner table again. I saw him in light, joy, and peace, and that made me happy. Then I saw him as a scared little boy, I saw someone who had been taught that he needs to, above all else, "be a good boy." He needed to do that regardless of how he felt or what he felt, and then the clarity once again stopped me in my tracks.

"Oh my gosh," I said aloud, even though no one was there. *He needed to ask me to marry him in order to be honorable about how we were spending our time together. He wanted to show up in honor to my family, and the best way he knew how was to ask them for my hand in marriage. And now, the only honorable thing he feels he can do is once again, pledge to marry me even though he doesn't want to marry me.*

Hundreds of chickadees startled me as they took off in flight, soaring across the mountain. It was gorgeous, a thousand lotus petals in flight in front of me, and so was this new way of seeing, just gorgeous.

Garrison, who I now saw as light, joy, and peace, so badly wanted to be and be seen as a good boy. He wanted this so much that he had, like I had done so many times, disconnected from how he felt and what he thought in order to focus on behaving in a way where he will "measure up" to what he thinks good is. This realization seemed to align with my sister's observation of him, that it was so important that he be seen and heard for his "good thoughts and deeds." He needed the validation because he fundamentally did not believe that he was "light, joy, and peace and that his sinlessness is guaranteed by God."

Then, I realized that I could only recognize this in Garrison because I do it as well. I have such a ridiculous need to be right; such a need to come off as the one who took the higher road, and I do this without being authentic. I reason away what I really feel and believe so that I come off looking good. I wanted to throw up at the thought of myself.

---

4   Baron Baptiste. Foundations in Teacher Training Workshop, Park City, Utah.

But then, I remembered, I am taking responsibility for ending this relationship. I am the one who is coming off as over-reacting to his announcement and looking as if I made a decision in fear instead of love. And I am making this decision as my authentic self. I don't want to marry Garrison. I don't want to live with him. I do want to be friends with him, and maybe one day I will be able to do that. But I don't need to see him when he wants to see me in a failed attempt to prove him wrong about my inability to become friends right now. I don't want to be friends right now. Right now, I don't want to see him again because he reminds me of what I need to remember about myself. Holy shit; now that is a lesson that I needed to learn.

Three doves scurried out from the bushes and across the rocks. I looked up at the sky, not sure if it was going to rain more or whether the sun would shine. I looked back down, no sign of the doves or the quails. I smiled and repeated my amended mantra all the way back down the mountain: "Light and joy and peace abide in you and in all beings. Your sinlessness is guaranteed by God. Connect your self to your Self. The answer to how is yes."

15   Forgiveness Gratitude

"Thank you so much, Garrison. I am so grateful to you for taking the time to meet up with us just before you fly out of town. You are so thoughtful." I actually couldn't believe the genuine gentleness and holy love that were flowing from me as I spoke these words. I never thought I would be sitting around a table at Sea World with my sisters, drinking crappy, overpriced margaritas, and looking across the table toward Garrison. We were having a last-minute catch-up chat five months after I slid the engagement ring toward him across the table at my favorite Italian restaurant.

I couldn't believe the peace that was filling my soul as I listened to him tell us what he had been up to for the last five months. How the "low-profile" life he had chosen was enriching his spirit and how his increased time spent in solitude was bringing him great peace and joy. He did seem to be genuinely well, and I loved how his initial somber spirit lightened immensely the more time he spent with my sisters and me. It was a true gift for all of us. As the catch-up conversation died down, I found myself praying to the Holy Spirit for wisdom in knowing just what to say and to whom, and then it just came out.

"Garrison," the soft and gentle voice that announced his name startled me, as that voice was so not my usual M.O. I guess it startled everyone as I felt everyone's eyes examining me closely for what was to come next. "Garrison," I said again, my voice still surprising me with its gentleness. "I want to apologize to you. I want to apologize to you for not being in a place where I could allow you the space to change your mind about marrying me without my making up some goofy story about it all."

Soft cleansing tears began to stream down my face. I was aware that I was the only one crying at the table. It seemed that I was not making much sense to anyone. So I explained.

I explained that what I had learned from studying A Course in Miracles (ACIM) was that I had apparently come up with a need to make up stories about things that I didn't fully understand. In other words, rather than recognizing that everything is love or a cry for love, I had chosen to live most of my life making up stories about why this happened or why that happened or blah, blah, blah. (At least that is what I sounded like to me, hopefully I made more sense to them.) I apologized to Garrison and my sisters for making up a story, for creating drama over his decision to change his mind. My drama creation created a lot of heartache for a lot of people. When all I really was called to do was kiss Garrison on the cheek and say, "Good on you, darling, for knowing what you believe serves the greatest good. I support you in that, and I will be fine. We are all connected. There are no mistakes or coincidences. When we think, speak, and then act out of our greatest good, all of us benefit."

We were all crying now. Apparently, the intended message inspired by the Holy Spirit had been delivered and had been heard. I felt lighter and more joyful in that moment than I had in a long time. We all clasped hands around the table and offered a prayer of gratitude for Garrison, for my sisters, for my life, and for the beautiful lessons our presence for each other brought us. As we dried our cleansing tears and returned to our teasing of each other, I glanced across the table toward Garrison. Our eyes met and I mouthed a "thank you" to him so as not to interrupt the story one of my sisters was now telling.

He smiled back at me. And in his smile, I saw forgiveness. I saw his forgiveness of me for creating drama over his changed mind, and I felt forgiveness of myself for having not been able to show up in a space that provided Garrison room to grow, room to show up differently than what I had wanted him to be for me. I was beaming now, beaming out a light of everlasting gratitude.

16 Belong to YOU?

Driving home from my *A Course in Miracles* (ACIM) discussion group, I found myself reflecting on the lesson that we had discussed in class. Earlier that week, I had been struggling with the desire to have a special guy in my life. I kept telling God that I was sure a special guy could help alleviate some of my day-to-day burdens so that I could focus more on my spiritual studies, and I had bargained with God, promising that a special guy could also help coach me in my spiritual journey.

This recent request to God was a step up from a conversation I had had with a friend just two weeks prior, when I had convinced myself that all I really needed was a warm body beside me in bed, someone that would clean up after himself. After her exclamation that what I had described was a cat, I decided to add on to the list of my desires. However, immediately upon adding the criteria that he must also be heterosexual, single, and unattached to another woman, particularly his mother, while also having a paying job, I was introduced to another awakening.

The earlier Sunday ACIM study group discussed that we were not to pray for what we want; rather, we were to focus on the cause of the desire and pray for peace and, in essence (or at least as I understood it), the removal of the desire. As such, we could see our desires and choose to focus on seeing them all differently; we could choose to focus on the source of the desire and thus move toward a focus on the creation of love and joy that would, in essence, remove all desire from our lives.

All of these teachings, while beautiful and I am sure meaningful, remained over my head, as all I could think about today (and the five days prior to this day), as I drove home from the study group, was that perhaps the cause of the desire for this special guy was an innate and ever growing need to have sex with someone special. I had become so horny in my current state of abstinence that I was staying home at night for fear I might literally jump on some guy walking by me. He then would surely think I was a nut case, and my chance at having this need met would end in humility. I was convinced that humility and horniness, while both starting with "h," did not go together.

As I completed my prayer, asking the Holy Spirit to help me see this ever growing desire for sex within a special relationship in a different light, perhaps in a light where I could focus on the peace, love, and joy of God rather than the fleeting moment of ecstasy that came from a roll in the hay, my phone rang.

It was my delightful little friend Leanna, calling me to see if I wanted to go out dancing that evening. "No," I emphatically exclaimed. "I can't."

She immediately became concerned.

"Oh, are you not feeling well? Are your legs not cooperating today?"

While I was experiencing significant pain in my legs, they were working quite well.

"No," I explained, "it is not that. I am so horny that I can't go out. I might jump some poor innocent bystander."

Leanna burst into laughter. "Since when are men who go dancing at nightclubs poor innocent bystanders?"

"Hey now," I replied in a voice that was attempting to defend the world, "we don't go to our dance hangout looking to get laid, and I want to keep it that way."

"All right, all right," she gave in reluctantly. We chatted about the date she had last night for a few minutes longer. Then I hung up and walked into an ice cream parlor. My plan was to distract myself from my desire by purchasing a very large amount of chocolate ice cream.

As the gal behind the counter completed what she surely thought must have been an order for my family of six, I looked down at my phone—a terrible habit I had gotten into whenever I had even two seconds to wait on service providers. I saw that I had four texts that had come in. One number had no name associated with it, and the text simply said, "Did you get it?" I assumed it was from one of my students who had e-mailed me an assignment and wanted to make sure I knew to check my e-mail for it; however, there was no name signed. The text just said, "Did you get it?" Not thinking anymore about it, I reached for my tub of chocolate ice cream, assured the kind young server that there was no need for a take home lid, grabbed a spoon, and headed out the door. I plopped down on one of the adorable little wicker chairs outside the shop and looked down at my phone again.

The same number had now sent a picture. *Oh, how fun,* I thought to myself. *Someone is enjoying this gorgeous day and sent me a picture.* I opened the photo and dropped my tub of ice cream.

"Holy shit!" I screamed, startling the people outside the ice cream parlor. They rushed to aid me, thinking that my starving family of six surely would be angry with me for dumping their tub of ice cream onto the concrete.

"It's okay, it's okay," I exclaimed as I shoved my phone back into its holster. "I, uh, I mean, they didn't need all these calories anyway." One dear gentleman offered to replace my tub of ice cream, commenting that the kids would really be disappointed. I smiled, not having the heart to admit that it was all for me right now to eat in one sitting, so that I could go home and better focus on my work. I just thanked him and assured him it would all be fine.

After cleaning up the mess on the concrete, I ran to the car and looked at my phone. Yup, I was not seeing things. Someone had texted me a photo of a penis. I was shocked. I stared at it for longer than should be advised. But I seriously wanted to know if I recognized it. I didn't. So then I thought, this has to be a joke. Who did I mention that I was horny to recently? Who would think this was funny? I immediately called Leanna back and challenged her.

"You would never believe what I just got!" I declared, rather annoyed, into my phone.

"What?" she exclaimed innocently, so innocently that I realized she couldn't have put anyone up to this. (She does live in a neighborhood where there are a lot of horny men, so it is not like she would have to go far to find someone willing to play this practical joke.) I told her the story of what I had just discovered on my phone, and she burst out laughing. I was able to drive all the way home before she stopped laughing.

"Well," she chided, "does it look familiar?"

"No," I said. "I have really studied it, and I have no idea who it belongs to." With that, she began to laugh aloud again; she laughed so long that I had to plug in my phone so the battery would last long enough for us to finish the phone call. "This is serious, Leanna," I exclaimed. "Who would have sent me this? This is kind of freaky."

She calmed down a little and then stated, "Well, maybe you should print it off and bring it to the dance club tonight and ask the regulars there if it belongs to them." With that, we both cracked ourselves up with the idea of our going around with the photo, asking random men if this belonged to them.

Finally, coming back to a semblance of sanity, I ended the phone call and looked down at my phone. I quite frankly was now beginning to get more than concerned. What freak sent me this? I chose not to give in to fear but to return to my earlier ACIM lessons of the day and of the previous week. Had I been so horny that I manifested this craziness? What was the source of this anyway? I began to feel a bit of fear taking hold of my body.

Shaking myself for a moment and choosing not to give into fear, I prayed to the Holy Spirit, asking for help to see this all differently. In that moment, I glanced down at my phone to see that a new text had come in from the same number; the person was apologizing, as he had the wrong number. I burst into laughter and praise at the same moment. I found myself thanking the Holy Spirit for the divine intervention, yet

I knew I had more work to do. I still wanted to understand the source of my desire, so I returned to prayer.

"Holy Spirit, please help me understand the source of this desire," I prayed as earnestly as I could, but before I could finish the full request, a thought came to my mind. I was sitting back in Dan's living room. Several of us, all good friends, were sitting on his floor, and we were listening to his new girlfriend's life story. She was telling us about the spiritual conversations that she had had while stripping and that she continued to have in the bars where she is a bartender. She was explaining to us that she had learned more about God and love in these venues than she did in church. At the time she was sharing these things, I was perplexed. I couldn't understand how someone could learn more about love in a strip joint than in a church. However, now, in this moment, I was no longer confused.

I had just realized that my craving for sex with a special guy was because I was craving a union with God. I had read in several books by many authors that they felt that the act of lovemaking with a committed partner was as close as our human minds could understand what union with God was really like. In this moment, in my kitchen, holding my little phone after having deleted the photo of a stranger's penis, and looking down at the chocolate ice cream splashes on my leg, I realized that my craving for sex with a special guy was nothing more than a confused craving for my union with God. That would explain why Dan's sweet new girlfriend felt that she had better conversations about who God is in strip joints; the folks there must have been seeking union with God and confusing sex with their desire to be one with God.

As I looked into the source of my craving, and as I acknowledged and accepted it for what I understood it to be, my craving evaporated. In that moment, there was truly nothing more that I desired than to be one with my God, to go home and to sit on his lap and have his arms wrapped around me. I had thought that desire could be met by simply having sex with a special guy. I prayed that I would never have that misunderstanding again.

17 Compassionate Dating

"I don't know, Marilee," Elisa declared as she slid her half-eaten plate of enchiladas away from her and peered through her long, black, flirtatious curls. She was grinning an extra ornery grin. "I think you should write a book on how to compassionately break up with men." With that comment, Laura started laughing but ended up choking on the rather large bite she had taken of the carne asada burrito she had just earlier been only staring at. While rushing to aid Laura, my conversation with Elisa didn't miss a beat.

"So, I should quit the book I am working on now and write a different one?" I inquired, my face looking rather annoyed by the thought of trying to find time away from my regular job to think about writing yet another book. My face contorted even more as I replied, "Yeah, right Elisa, that will look really good on my academic CV. I'll get kicked out of the academy for sure if I try to write that; besides, what would it even be about?"

Laura had managed to swallow the rather large piece of burrito that had been choking her with, of course, absolutely no real help from Elisa and me; she cleaned her palate with a swirl of her diet Pepsi and piped in.

"I know, I know," she exclaimed with enthusiasm that caught Elisa and me off guard. I glanced down at Laura with the sudden realization that she no longer needed our assistance and wondered how a person who had just been choking on a huge bite of carne asada burrito could be so enthusiastic and clearly articulate right now. My thoughts didn't interrupt Laura's enthusiasm as she continued, "You could write about the time I got an extra order of garlic fries so as to dissuade my date from even thinking about kissing me, let alone asking me out again. Or how about the time I ate a whole box of Altoids, feeling so nervous about the first kiss with a guy I didn't want to kiss, that I ended up getting sick and throwing them up, which resulted in an early end to the disastrous date? Oh, then there was the time I texted you the SOS message so you could call me fifteen minutes into the date with a fake emergency to get me out of the date."

I was grimacing with the memory of these stories as Elisa was holding her sides with laughter.

"No, no, Laura ..." Elisa's speech was broken by the snorts that always come out when she laughs uncontrollably. "We are talking about compassionate break-ups, not date escapes."

"I don't know," I said reflectively, interrupting Elisa by handing her a glass of water. I was afraid she would start choking like Laura was earlier. "I think something called *Date Escapes* might actually be helpful and thus get read as opposed to something called *Compassionate Break-Ups*. I think we would have more material too."

Laura and I continued to laugh at this idea, but Elisa settled into a sobering voice.

"I am serious, Marilee." Her tender yet earnest tone caused me to look up from my taco salad that I had been wrestling with for about twenty minutes. *How do you actually eat one of these things gracefully when they are in those deep fried bowls anyway?* I peered into Elisa's deep brown eyes. Was that a tear in her eye from laughter, or was she about to cry? The sight of it pulled me back into a place of sensitivity.

"I am sorry, Elisa, I am listening."

Elisa explained the concern that she had entering the dating field after her seventeen-year marriage had ended. She and her husband worked hard to end their marriage as lovingly as they had begun it. I admired how they moved through their divorce, and oddly enough, I felt honored to be part of the loving conversations they shared. I was encouraged by how they continued to love and honor each other, something I did not do when both of my marriages ended. Elisa and her former husband had truly moved through their separation in love, honor, and admiration as they ended their marriage commitment to each other.

I stared at Elisa admiringly. She was gorgeous and bright, with a delightful energy and matching personality. As she spoke of her dating trepidations, I could see in her eyes the memory of the pain she felt she had caused her husband by choosing to end the marriage. And I could see that she had no desire to repeat endings of relationships in the dating arena, knowing that she may once again cause someone pain.

Laura also watched in silence and then quickly averted her eyes, looking back down at her barely eaten burrito. I asked Laura if she was okay. She sipped on her diet Pepsi before peering up through her long blonde hair. She didn't respond. I saw in her tender blue eyes what was surely another tear. She no doubt was recalling her horrible divorce and the two icky dating break-ups that followed when she returned to the dating game.

Good grief, I thought to myself. *How can we go from laughing our asses off in one moment to nearly bawling our eyes out in the other?* Smiling, I remembered that was why I adored these two. We had lots of moments like that, and those moments made my life so rich, so alive, and so amazing.

Confused by my smile, Laura wiped her tears and innocently inquired, "What are you thinking, Marilee?"

Not answering with the truth of what I was actually thinking, I decided to try to make them laugh again, so I recounted some stories we had all shared.

"Okay, so would you want the book to talk about how I met that one annoying guy at our dance club? Remember? We thought he was just a regular, nice guy, so we were all engaged in great conversation and fun dancing, but then he drank too much and started to get clingy, that gross kind of clingy. He wouldn't stop, so I replied to him as compassionately as I could, 'I know we are all connected; I know we are all one; and therefore, you are the part of me whose sorry ass I am going to leave hanging in this bar while the rest of me goes home with my girlfriends?'"

That did it; they were laughing again. And Laura was energized to chime into the conversation.

"Or how about that other time, when that guy kept creepily following you around at the wine tasting event and you said, 'I read recently that when I come across something to which I cannot respond in love, I simply should just turn away.' And then you did the marching band three-point turn around and walked away."

They were both laughing now. The trick had worked; sharing stories of my silly adventures got them laughing again. However, now my face was somber as I reflected back upon those stories. That wasn't compassionate behavior I had exhibited; that was ego. And ego invites ego; ego reflects ego. There is no true love compassion in ego. While I was happy to see that Elisa and Laura were entertaining themselves with more memories, more silly stories of how we attempted to be loving and compassionate and failed miserably, the realization that in thinking I was acting in love, but discovering that I was still acting with ego was a hard pill to swallow. Would I choke next? I sipped some water and took a moment to pray.

I prayed a prayer I had learned from studying ACIM; I simply asked the Holy Spirit how I might see this all differently. As I was engaged in my request, Elisa and Laura noticed that I was no longer participating verbally. Being the beautiful, encouraging souls that they are, they simply went into prayer themselves, the same prayer I was praying, for we were all studying the Course.[5]

After a moment, we looked at each other and smiled. I invited them to share what had come to them. They wanted me to share first, so I explained that in reflecting on how I would behave if I truly were trying to end a date or even an encounter with someone in compassion, I would simply go no further than recommending what we had already

---

5   A Course in Miracles.

read in the Course. All we have to remember is that we are all One in Christ, One in God, or One in whatever you want to call your God. If I simply remember that what I am doing to this person I encounter or to this date, I am doing to myself, then that would certainly mean that I would end the date with compassion. "The book on compassionate date ending has already been written, you guys; it is called the Course."

I sat back, smiling contently, until my wiser friend, Elisa, spoke up. "Yeah, well, what do you do when the guy you just met or the one you just ended your date with didn't read it? What do you do then?" she further challenged.

Laughing aloud, I knew what she was talking about. I had recently ended a dating relationship with Wyatt. And Wyatt did not want to have anything to do with ACIM; that was okay with me. ACIM, after all, is not a religion, and I had found its principles of love applicable to all religions, philosophies, and spiritual practices. When my laughter died down, I reminded Elisa and Laura that they had helped me with that compassionate and love-filled ending, for they coached me into a space of love in the ending of that relationship. They had reminded me to own only what I believe and to not judge Wyatt for where he was in his journey and what his expressed needs conveyed. They reminded me not to judge him or judge myself for feeling that I was no longer showing up as my best self in this relationship. Through their support and much prayer, I was able to reflect love and send out love through the ending process, even when Wyatt was not in a place of love or compassion. It really had worked.

Elisa paused for a moment, and a smile began to creep onto her gorgeous, shining face, as she confessed, "Yes, the book has already been written."

As we paid our bills and got ready to depart, I stopped for a moment to jot down a reminder note for myself. I guess we just needed to remind each other that even when the guy is showing up in his best dressed ass-hole suit, we can still choose love. We can, as Marianne Williamson[6] suggests, picture their harsh words turning into roses and

---

6   Marianne Williamson. *A Return to Love: Reflections on the Principles of the Course in Miracles.* New York: HarperCollins, 1992.

falling at our feet. We can picture our face on theirs; we can think of how we might need to be treated with compassion even if we are angry or hurt. And we can remind ourselves that in our darkest hours or in the darkest hours of another, all there is is love; everything else is just a cry for love.

18　Maintaining Identity

"People are going to think you are crazy; you know that, don't you?" Patty exclaimed, stopping only for a moment on our arduous hike to catch her breath and to make certain I had received the intentionality of her message. I laughed so heartily I had to stop walking as well and bend over to catch my breath.

"Yes, I know," I managed to reply through gasps of air. "I am looking forward to being called 'crazy.'"

As I continued to laugh with my head dangling between my legs, I began to sense that Patty no longer thought this was the least bit funny. Slowly, I raised my torso and then my head, wiping away wind-swept tears in my eyes, and examined her expression. Her furrowed brow and partial frown jolted me out of my laughter.

"Are you okay, Patty?" I inquired with sincere concern for the well-being of my friend.

"Honestly, Marilee," she said emphatically, moving forward in her fast-paced stride once more, "I am worried. I don't think you know who you are, and now you want to go off and write this book and ..."

As serious and as loving as my friend Patty was being, I couldn't help myself. I burst into loud, obnoxious laughter again as I ran to catch up with her; my obnoxious laughter drowned out the rest of her loving reprimand. Trying to gather my legs and my wits about me, I could tell that my laughter had not been received as I intended. Of course it had not; I had completely insulted my beautiful friend.

"I am so sorry, Patty," I apologized. "I really am."

Patty looked down at the muddy path on which we were hiking. She was shaking her head in utter disgust. After what felt like an eternity, she finally stopped shaking her head and looked back up at me. The partial frown was now replaced by a distinct and rather pronounced scowl. "What are you doing, Marilee? Who are you? You can't be successful in your field and tell people you respect that the way they do most of the things they do at work no longer makes sense to you. Seriously, do you even know who you are?"

This was one of those moments where the logic part of your mind was supposed to kick in and respond by discounting all your foolishness that you earlier expressed. This was one of those moments when you were supposed to tell yourself to apologize, retract all you said, and get yourself back into line with who you are supposed to be and how you are supposed to be behaving. Apparently, however, on that day, that part of my mind was, well, on vacation. For instead of responding as I once most likely would have, I burst into even louder and even more obnoxious laughter.

My eyes were tearing even more; I was hysterically laughing, and I was filled with joy as I did so. My poor friend, Patty, looked even more bewildered than ever, and I saw her glance down at her phone to determine whether she had cell service, thus considering dialing 911 to have me put away once and for all. That sight made me even more amused.

As my laughter died down, my speech slowly returned. "Beautiful Patty," I began. "I feel your love and I recognize your concern. I am so deeply blessed to have a friend like you who cares so deeply about my well-being. I don't mean to offend you or disrespect you by my laughter. It is just that, well, I no longer want to pretend that I know who I am."

Patty's face showed increasing signs of perplexity, so I continued on with my ramblings, hoping her facial muscles would soon find relief.

I explained to her that I had recently come to realize that in clinging to my ego-identified self, I never made space for renewal, for expansion, for reinvention, for spirit to re-create or cocreate a new "reality" for me. Rather, I just dug myself deeper into a trench that I called "myself." I further explained that in trying to hold on so dearly to who I thought I was or who I wanted others to believe I was, I never risked the challenge of just being, of just experiencing, of just discovering. I was finding no room for mindfulness in my battle to maintain my ego-identified self. Therefore, I no longer wanted to be identified as "me." Rather, I was inviting what I understood to be "me" to be open to learning from others and ultimately to exemplify the joy and love that I understood we are all called to be. I really, more than anything, wanted to lose myself, lose my ego, and lose my identity. I wanted to not know who I am.

While Patty listened earnestly and while her face did relax, I could tell she still thought I was insane. I didn't have to read her mind; when she realized my monologue had ended, she affirmed this belief to me. "Everyone is going to think you lost it; everyone is going to call you crazy."

I laughed aloud again. We were at the beginning of our conversation once more. *It amazes me how so many things move in circles*, I thought to myself, still giggling at the return of our initial conversation.

Smiling more widely than the path upon which we were walking, I flung my arm around Patty's shoulder and pulled her closely in toward my left side. The joy that radiated into my arm that reached for Patty created such force that it almost knocked us both off of our feet and into the muddy puddle on the right side of the path. The awkward move caused her to smile and wriggle out of my hold. She stopped once again and looked deeply into my eyes. "Well, this is going to be interesting to watch," she smirked.

Delighted by the sparkle that had returned to her Irish green eyes, my rejuvenated response was only another laugh. It was, after all, the expression that most resonated with what I understood my new "state of being" to now reflect: joy, pure unabashed and resounding joy. *Yes*, I thought to myself. This is going to be interesting to observe. It will be interesting to see how I am able to no longer identify with my ego, but learn to walk a journey that allows the old "me" to disappear as a new identity with love unfolds.

19 Dizziness and Giddiness

I read the words again as I sat at my kitchen counter. Reading my mail as I relaxed in my kitchen at the end of a long day of work was a daily routine I looked forward to doing. As I reread the words, my laughter bounced and echoed off the tile floors and the large wall of windows as if I had just yelled a big ole whoop at the bottom of the Grand Canyon. I couldn't believe my eyes. So, I read it a fourth time: "We have reviewed your claim for ambulance services and approved your hospitalization for dizziness and giddiness. Therefore, we will cover your ambulance transfer costs ..."

"Dizziness and giddiness?" I announced aloud to no one at all and began to laugh so hard, I nearly fell off the bar stool upon which I was seated at my kitchen counter. As the laughter turned to tears in my eyes, I recalled the scene in which I had to file an insurance claim to cover the ambulance ride I was reading about in the official insurance correspondence. It was an early autumn Monday afternoon, and I was at work. I was preparing to meet a colleague at the on-campus Starbucks to discuss his research agenda. I had arrived early for the meeting, so I stood in the long line and prepared to order my usual green tea soy latte, no classic, and no foam. The line was typically long, so I was thinking I should pull out the Blackberry from my hip holster to text my colleague to see if I could place his order. As I leaned forward to place my always-way-too-overloaded briefcase onto the floor between my legs and stood back up to reach for my Blackberry on my hip, I crumbled to the ground.

I had no warning. I simply fell to the floor like a building being demolished in such an orchestrated fashion that it fell perfectly straight down, no falling over to one side, just a simple crumbling of the foundation, a direct line down, directly down. I fell in a heap right on top of the briefcase that looked as if it was ready to give birth; the same briefcase that only seconds earlier I had so carefully placed between my legs.

I didn't panic. I seriously thought that I may have been dreaming and all I had to do was awaken to realize that I was dreaming. I began to have that dream conversation where you coach yourself to awaken when I heard a very different voice; it was a very concerned male voice, and it was coming from behind me. The voice asked me if I was all right. I looked forward and realized the line had moved, yet I hadn't moved at all. This was so unlike me. I walk and drive like I am from Boston. I allow no space between the next person and me, whether I am waiting in line on foot, or whether I am in a car. So, this clearly wasn't a dream, it was a nightmare.

At this time and in this moment, I didn't look back at the voice, I looked forward. And I noticed that there was space now for three people between me and the person in front of me. While I panicked in that moment, because I realized someone could easily cut in front of me, I also realized that I was unable to move at all. *Yup,* I thought to myself, *I have to be dreaming—this has to be a nightmare. I can't move anything but my head and neck.* Giving into the fact that I could only move my head and neck, I looked toward the voice. I wasn't sure what I would see. Maybe it would be George Clooney. After all, I was convinced I was dreaming, so it could be George Clooney. Yet, if this was a nightmare, it was probably, well, somebody else. This was all just too weird.

"Uh," I stuttered, looking up to the voice that resonated from above, "I think you may want to go around me. I can't seem to move." I heard the voice again, and now, I could see his face. It was a young man

I didn't recognize and who was now bending over me. He repeated, "Are you okay?"

Now ... I was really feeling panic as I couldn't seem to awaken from this dream, and I really couldn't move, and more importantly, I had lost all concept of how many spaces were in between me and the person in front of me in the Starbucks line.

"I can't seem to move," I repeated, feeling the panic increase even more.

"Dr. Bresciani?" I heard a familiar voice behind me, but I couldn't turn to see who it was. The person with the voice moved in front of me, and I could see it was one of the students in our master's program. My panic eased when I felt her warmth and love radiate toward me.

"Hey you!" I smiled, delighted to see her. "How are you?"

She returned my smile with an even brighter and warmer smile.

"I am fine, Dr. Bresciani, but how are you? Are you okay?"

"Ya know," I responded slowly and carefully, still trying to move, "I don't think I am. I better call someone to come get me." When my brain told my arm and hand to reach for my phone, my arm responded and swung in the direction of my hip, but my hand didn't grab the phone. Rather, it just hung by my side. "Hmm ...," I said, still feeling as if I was observing myself in a dream. "That is weird." I felt as if I was suspended in time.

The fabulous student didn't miss a beat. Trained to react in crisis situations, she grabbed my Blackberry out of my holster and asked who she should call. I told her who to call while simultaneously realizing that I couldn't get control of my movements and wasn't sure what I should do next. My mind was in a debate about whether I was dreaming all of this and wondering why I couldn't wake up and take back control of the situation. While I sat there, or rather crumpled there, in a daze, the student took control of the situation. She was amazing. She was completing a 911 call, filling out a Starbucks accident report, trying to call our program administrative assistant to let her know that I wouldn't be in class later that afternoon, and getting me moved out of the Starbucks line. I think there were about eight spaces now between the next person and me.

The next thing I felt was pain underneath my armpits as two very tall young men lifted me out of the line and proceeded to lay me on the floor. I wasn't very helpful. I felt I had no control of anything below my waist and very little control of my arms. *This is so weird*, I kept thinking.

I was trying to make light of it, telling myself that surely I was dreaming all of this and very soon I would awaken and laugh at it all. I remember looking into the eyes of some very handsome firemen and telling them, "Really? Don't even think about asking me what year it is or what day it is, I never know that information. However, I can tell you that I am late for my one o'clock appointment and I have a 2:30 after that, followed by class at four o'clock, so whatever you need to fix in this body, you better do it quickly. I got work to do."

Apparently, that smart-ass comment, followed by several others, including me reciting aloud that "Nothing real can be threatened. Nothing unreal exists. So, this must not be real,"[7] prompted the diagnosis of "dizziness and then the giddiness."

How weird is that? I thought as I leaned back on my stool at my kitchen counter. I didn't respond as they had expected. Rather, I was reciting what I had learned in the Course. I was convinced that my collapse in the Starbucks was the result of some elaborate story my subconscious was trying to tell me. And even though I was fully aware of what I was not able to do, I was also fully aware that I was dreaming and that this would pass as soon as I decided I no longer needed to learn the lesson that I was to learn.

I remembered lying in the emergency room bed with the usual battery of tests being done yet again. I remembered joking with the hospital staff and the perplexed looks on people's faces, wondering why I would be laughing when I couldn't feel my legs. I kept repeating, "Nothing real can be threatened. Nothing unreal exists. Herein lies the peace of God." In this moment, it all came to this. This belief allowed me to laugh, this belief allowed me to joke with folks, and this belief brought the medics to write on my ambulance transfer … "dizziness and giddiness."

---

7   A Course in Miracles, Introduction.

I leaned forward in my stool and set the letter back down on the granite counter. I admired my countertops for a moment. I was so glad I had invested in the granite to replace the broken tiles that wee there when I purchased the place. I stared at the patterns in the granite and imagined the strength of the creature from whom this beautiful piece was pried; the beautiful piece that had made its way into my home, now offering beauty and groundedness to those who saw that within it as they took food and wine from the resting place upon it.

The granite countertop looked and felt very real to me, but that collapse in the Starbucks didn't. Why is that? Why does the window look like an illusion but the tile floors appear to be so solid? Why does the white orchid appear to be surreal and the water in my glass appear so very real? "Nothing real can be threatened. Nothing unreal exists. Herein lies the peace of God." I repeated the phrase again. "Nothing real can be threatened. Nothing unreal exists." I pushed myself away from the countertop and began to laugh at all the crazy stories that I make up about things that happen to me within my day-to-day life; they take so much of my time and energy. *No wonder I was committed for dizziness and giddiness*, I thought to myself, laughing. How can I not become dizzy from the insane pace in which I live and then become giddy when I attempt to laugh it all away?

"Nothing real can be threatened. Nothing unreal exists. Herein lies the peace of God." *These are words to live by,* I thought to myself. *This will ensure that the next time I am committed, it will only read, "She was giddy."*

20 Holy Intimacy

"Woo, that is a mess in there," Allen announced as he continued to lay his hand upon my abdomen with the gentleness and care that can only belong to a seasoned healer.

"You're telling me," I winced, laying flat on my back on top of his acupuncture table. My eyes were closed tightly, and tears were making their way down the sides of my face, falling gently onto the white paper that lined the table. I was in a lot of pain today, not the kind where you are doubled over and throwing up, nor the kind where you crumble to your feet and someone has to hold you up just so you can lie on your back to catch your breath. This was just regular pain, yet it was the kind that keeps you from fully focusing on what you really need to be focusing on; like the stuff that earns you your salary.

Allen took awhile longer. I could feel his hand, his magical healing hand I called it, as it rested on my unzipped jeans, which only slightly revealed my purple lace panties underneath. My mother taught me a long time ago that you should always wear panties that are nice and clean, in case you ever get in a car accident. That saying never made sense to me. After all, if I got in a car accident, I am confident that the last thing I would be thinking of is whether my panties were nice and clean. What did make sense to me as a single woman, however, is that you should always wear sexy panties just in case. Well, in case you had to unzip your jeans just enough to reveal a wee bit of your panties for a handsome healer to feel your energy flow blockage in your abdomen.

"What do you think is going on down there?" he asked me in a very compassionate tone.

I resisted my first reactive response, which was, "Aren't I paying you to tell me what is going on down there?" Instead, my eyes, which were previously only sprinkling tears, now began to feed a steady waterfall. "I continue to struggle with a need for intimacy and companionship and a desire for a holy relationship." That was all I could get out before the dam that was holding back the tears broke. I was in a full-fledged waterfall.

Allen didn't flinch; he didn't react. Instead, I heard him take a deep meditative breath. I felt holy love flow from his hand onto my abdomen, through my jeans and my purple lace panties, as he described to me in detail the seriously sad shape of my uterus and ovaries. Then, he breathed again and began to share his wisdom. I believe it was his selfless and ego-less sharing of his wisdom that kept me coming back to his office just as much, if not more, than his healing touch.

Allen began to share the lessons he had learned at a workshop he had attended earlier that month. He talked about how the facilitator said that sometimes we have to hold the holy and the profane within the same space. He spoke of the yin and the yang and the challenges of taking a dualistic way of thinking and moving it toward pure nondualism. He spoke once again to me of my warrior's desire to protect my playful child and how all that may just be exactly what I was experiencing in my body as my abdomen fought my heart.

Allen continued to share his wisdom as he carefully placed the acupuncture needles into my primary meridian. He asked me to imagine the release of the pressure I felt in my abdomen. He asked me to visualize it as if it was a gusher, coming up to my heart and pouring out of me in perfect love, rather than anger; pouring out of me in joy, rather than fear; pouring out of me in peace while my left hand held onto profanity and my right hand held onto the holy relationship. With that, Allen left the room so that I could move into my meditative state.

Yeah, well, all that was beautiful and it was so not helpful in stopping the tears, which were now making me wonder whether anyone had been treated for dehydration due to too much crying. Furthermore, I had acupuncture needles in my hands, so no way in hell was I going to try to wipe away my tears for fear I would look like Edward Scissorhands before I got off the table.

Deciding not to worry about dehydration or how crusty my mascara was going to look *(why don't I just break down and buy waterproof mascara?)*, I returned to the images Allen asked me to consider as I lay on the table for my treatment. Hold the profane and the holy within the same space.

That was my problem. I had never told Allen about my sexual history. Maybe he already knew, but how did he know? Could he feel the turmoil in my abdomen? *I couldn't do it,* I immediately said to myself. I couldn't hold images of being engaged in forceful sex and lustful sex and sex to try to win a companion and sex engaged within a loving, committed union within the same sphere. I couldn't hold what felt like the profane and the holy within the same space. I began to feel like I was suffocating by simply trying to hold those thoughts within the space of my body.

"Yowza!" I cried out.

It felt as if my ovaries were going to push right out of my skin. My scream brought Allen rushing back into the room. He wisely didn't ask how it was going, for fear no doubt that I would yank the needles out of my body and try to stick them in him. He just moved peacefully and gently toward the table and laid his hands over my third eye. He coached me about my breathing; he coached me into a more peaceful state, before he asked me whether I was okay.

In response to his question, I oddly found myself smiling. I explained to him that I was grateful for this abdominal pain. For without it, I would not have known I was having such a struggle with what I felt was a conflict between a desire for intimacy and a desire for a holy relationship. Now I was laughing, as I told him about the lecture I had shared with my students the night before. Inspired by Deepak Chopra's

The Soul of Leadership, I was using information from his first chapter on looking and listening to explain to my research methodology students that deep inquiry requires them to go beyond the use of their analytical mind; it requires them to engage in being mindful of the data their body is providing them as well as the data their emotions are providing them.

I shared all this with Allen, and we both found ourselves laughing in gratitude for the gifts of awareness that the body can share with us, if only we are willing to listen. Allen adjusted the acupuncture needles and invited me once again to move back into the guided imagery and relaxation that earlier had failed. I found myself in a different place. I saw my body on a white table. I saw my warrior on my left side and my innocent, playful child on my right. I saw an open empty tube within my body. The blood in my abdomen was flowing freely toward my heart. Out of my mouth poured heart-shaped droplets of blood that flowed onto the floor and through the cracks in the old wooden floor planks. As I visualized this, I found myself breathing easily, and I felt no pain, no pressure.

I could see that the love, in the form of heart-shaped droplets of blood, which was oozing from my mouth was nurturing the ground beneath the table. I could see that the warrior was watching the profane, and he was ensuring that while it was within the sphere of my body, it would not be allowed to harm the little girl merrily playing on my right with joyful innocence and unconditional love. And the little girl? She knew nothing of lust, of force, of desire; she was fully engaged in holy, everlasting, unconditional love, peace, and joy.

21 Connected Life

I awakened to see the sun shining through the sheers of my hotel room. *What a glorious day*, I thought to myself as I rolled over to check the time on the alarm clock. It was earlier than I actually wanted to get up; however, the convincing rays streaming through the eggshell shears provided all the motivation I needed to literally roll myself out of bed. I told myself I would do my morning meditation in the mountains, there could be no better place. I heated a pot of water for tea and washed the sleep from my eyes.

In my morning readying process, I stopped just for a moment to read my ACIM daily lesson, and then I peeked one more time out the window to see how many layers of clothing I would need. I had never been in Estes Park, Colorado, in the winter, and I was not accustomed to cold weather. I was proud to be a southern girl with regard to my comfort level with living in warm weather. Gauging the temperature by the frost on the truck windows below in the hotel parking lot, I grabbed an extra layer as well as my camera and readied myself for my adventure in the Rocky Mountain National Park. "This was going to be an awesome day," I announced to the universe on my way out of my hotel room door.

And it was. Right up until the time I sat down for dinner.

Estes Park, Colorado, and the Rocky Mountain National Park have always been a place where I have felt my heart nurtured and my spirit awakened my entire life. It didn't matter whether I had vacationed there with my family as a child, or later camping with girlfriends, or the many times I had come to hike and climb with men I was dating. It didn't matter the company nor the context; it had always been a place of peace and restoration for me. It was a place where I truly understood in a soulful way that we are all one with the land and the sky and with each other.

This day started out no differently. Since I had never been to Estes Park in winter, I was not sure what to expect. It was gorgeous, as always, yet even more peaceful and serene than it was in the summer, with the hoards of people eager to take in its beauty. I felt I had the entire park to myself. I drove the snow-covered roads, stopping in the middle of the road to take pictures, feeling as if no one would even come upon me at all, and no one ever did.

As I snapped photos of rocks, trees, clouds, sky, mountains, and valleys, I would whisper, "We are all one," and I would feel these words resonate with every cell of my being. Even as the snows came across the mountains and I retreated into the village of Estes Park to stroll the streets, I could see the God in every person I encountered and feel the connection we had. "We are all one," I kept repeating. "We are all God, always, all of the time." I could really feel it.

I could feel this connection whether I entered a stylish boutique, where I couldn't even afford to buy a handkerchief, or popped into a shop that was filled with Buddhist prayer flags, wheels, and singing bowls. The latter shop was of particular interest. The proprietor of this shop, after discovering that I practiced meditation, insisted that I place a singing bowl on my head as he struck the side of it so that I could better meditate. All was going beautifully until he proceeded to strike the bowl repeatedly and with great force, at the point where the bowl rested directly atop my head. Concerned that this type of meditation would result in me either passing out or having a concussion, I gently grabbed the mallet in midair strike, pulled the bowl from my head, handed both bowl and mallet to him as I bowed to him, and backed out of the shop saying, "Namaste."

It was truly a glorious day. I found my eyes tearing at each encounter; I had never felt such a day where every encounter was so loving, so intense, so connected. Yes, this was the day I had. It was glorious, as I mentioned, until I went out for dinner.

Having grown to love the ACIM prayer, "Show me where you would have me go, what you would have me do, what you would have me say and to whom," I prayed this prayer as I headed out from my hotel that evening for my dinner. I was so hungry. I had only snacked all day because, as usual, I was caught up in the experience of the moment, and I had forgotten to tend to my fueling needs. So I was ready to eat. As I drove away from my hotel, I turned my rented four-wheel drive toward the village, personally desiring to commune more with the locals and have a hearty winter meal. Instead, I found myself driving across the valley and up the other side to a famous hotel for dinner.

This is odd, I thought to myself. *Why am I doing this? Why I am headed there when I really wanted to go elsewhere?* The historic hotel was gorgeous and the wait staff seemed accustomed to making sure everyone's needs were met beyond their initial expression. I felt like a princess as I was ushered into the dining room and seated at a corner that was quite, well, isolated from the rest of the guests. After all, I was alone, and everyone else in the restaurant was, well, with someone or with several people.

I played with stories in my head for just a moment. *Maybe they have mistaken me for a famous person and don't want me to be bothered by any fans. Or maybe they felt that since I was alone, I wanted to continue to be in a "lonely" physical place.* The wait staff couldn't have been more gracious and accommodating. The food and wine were fabulous. So why was I making a big deal out of being several feet away from the nearest table?

I no longer felt connected. I no longer felt like we were all one. Even from afar, as I studied all the guests' faces, I was telling myself, *We are all one. You are me and I am you. We are all God, all of the time.* Yet I felt so far away. What was I projecting into this situation that made me feel so disconnected? Surely it wasn't the hostess's fault. What was I seeing that was not really there?

I finished the last bite from my plate, took my last sip of wine, and paid the bill. It was a beautiful meal, the hotel was as elegant as had been described to me, and the staff again was beyond delightful. My senses were satisfied, yet I felt empty. How could that possibly be? I strolled into the cold night air and noticed that the clouds that had brought snow earlier had cleared. I could see the stars, and the moonlight revealed the snow on the peaks across the valley. "Just gorgeous, absolutely gorgeous," I said aloud as I stood in the middle of the parking lot to admire the beauty that had unfolded before me. *This will fill me back up*, I thought, yet the vastness of the sky and the majesty of the mountains only seemed to echo the emptiness I felt inside.

As I settled myself behind the wheel of the massive four-wheel drive, I stared at the dashboard as if looking for some type of indicator that would help me better understand why I was feeling so empty.

"Aw ...," I exclaimed aloud. "Seat heaters; that ought to do it. What a great invention!" I flipped the switch. My bum became instantly warm, but my soul did not. *Hmmm*, I wondered, *Why didn't that work?* Without praying my prayer, I headed toward the village, camera in tow, to snap some shots of the spectacular village white lights.

Jumping out of the truck, camera readied for action, I was bound and determined to change my thoughts about what I was feeling. This was gorgeous after all and very exciting, and who knows what pictures were ahead of me to snap? I looked forward to the encounters with beautiful souls I may likely yet have this evening. As I bounded out of the truck, camera in hand, and enthusiasm refueled, my snow boots hit the icy pavement with a reverberating thud. It was as if the sound was reminding me that I had not yet done the work that my thoughts had raised in the restaurant. "I'll tend to those thoughts later," I said to myself. It was time now to capture some magic with the camera.

As I found just the right shot, I smiled, aimed, focused, smiled even wider, and nothin'. The camera refused to cooperate. I didn't understand. I had recharged the battery before going to dinner, unloaded the memory card on my laptop, and adjusted the right lens before even placing it back into its protective bag. I had brought it into the restaurant with me so it would not get too cold. What was up? Getting colder by the moment trying to figure it all out, I looked back up at the sky and announced grudgingly to the stars, "Okay, okay, I will go back to my room and address this empty feeling like a, like a, like a woman."

Back in my toasty warm hotel room, I unfolded my yoga mat. I knew I would not practice yoga for the second time today. My full stomach was reminding me that that would be a bad idea. Instead, I lay upon my back on the yoga mat in the surrender pose. Savasana, sweet surrender. As I lay there, staring up at the popcorn ceiling, wondering if there was asbestos in that popcorn and wondering how wise it was to lie below it, I began my conversation with God and my conversation with myself. My first question was, *After such a glorious day of seeing you [God] in every living thing and nonliving thing (including the expensive purple handkerchief at the chi chi boutique), how is it that I can end the day feeling so alone just because of where I was seated in a restaurant? Holy Spirit, please help me see this differently.*

With that, the tears began to flow. I laughed a little at myself wondering whether this release was the gift of the little Buddhist man in the shop who whacked me over the head three times with the mallet; perhaps those are the kind of wake-up calls that God needs to provide me, literal whacks over the head. Or perhaps it was a release that came from simply taking the time to stop and ask the Holy Spirit for help to see this situation differently and then sincerely stop to listen.

I cried for what seemed like hours. In the crying, I saw past visions of me enjoying the park with all of those I so dearly loved, some who were still in this world but no longer in my life, some who have already transitioned out of this world, and some whom I love and who are still in my life but are now showing up in it in a different way, or rather I am showing up in their lives in a different way. In particular, I realized that I was missing Garrison, that I had really wanted to enjoy this place with him again as we had done before. I had wanted him to join me for dinner, but he wasn't there. And then I realized that he was still with me even though he was with me in a different way than I wanted him to be.

I recognized that I chose to see the place where I was seated in the restaurant as an isolated place, rather than a place where I could observe, listen, and feel. I chose to feel isolated because I was choosing separation. I was still just as connected to everyone in that room, but I chose not to feel it just because I was dining alone in a place often reserved for those who dined with another. My tears gave way to my laughter as I sat up with the realization that at any time, I could have asked to be seated somewhere else. I could have asked to have my meal moved to the bar, where I could sit and listen to others chatting away. I could have stepped out for a moment to call one of my fabulous friends and told her where I was and that I would be thinking of her as I enjoyed the meal, making me feel even more connected. I could have done a number of things, or I could have simply sat there and chose to see it all differently. Instead, I chose to feel separated.

ACIM teaches us to choose again. When we make a choice that causes us to feel separated from the divine, we should simply choose again. Sitting on my yoga mat in my hotel room with the popcorn ceiling, I chose to choose again. I am connected to all of those with whom I was sitting in the dining room tonight, even though we never made eye contact. We are all one, and whenever I feel all alone, all I have to do if I need aid is reach out to my Sangha of friends, albeit in newly made ones or ones that have been with me through thick and thin. I am not alone, I am never alone, and we are all connected all the time. We are all God all of the time.

22   Surrendering

"Donita, do you mind looking over my holiday letter to make sure it doesn't sound stupid before I send it out to friends and family?" I called across the coffee shop to my friend who was waiting to get us refills on our tasty hot beverages. Donita glanced back at me, looking over her shoulder with the expression of a fifteen-year-old who had just been embarrassed by her mother yelling, "I love you," across the high school parking lot after being dropped off on her first day of school. I saw Donita purse her lips and scowl at my request. I read that speechless expression as an affirmative. So, I did what only certifiably obnoxious friends do next. I yelled, "Thank you! I love you." To which she quickly exited the coffee queue and bee-lined for the bathroom in complete embarrassment. I smiled as I watched her race far away from me. *I really do love her,* I thought. And I returned to editing my holiday letter.

December 24

Merry Peace, Joy, Love, and Light!!!

Wow! 2010 was an amazing year! So many lessons were learned this year and I thank you for your part in making that all true for me.

Awakening!

It started with a work assignment and resulting retreat in Hawaii for my 45th birthday, where the message of our individual completeness was made evident. What so many of you had been trying to teach me for years was finally understood on the islands. That understanding opened up a whole new level of learning for me; learning that blossomed through avenues (Conversations with God readings, Meditation classes, Spiritual whatever they were classes, Visioning webinars, and long, long nights of discussions, meditation, and prayer) that I would have not been previously open to receiving. Awesome stuff! Thank you for being a part in my awakening.

Celebrating!

The late spring and summer brought many more celebrations of lessons learned and other avenues ventured. Again, many in which I would have never previously fully explored (yoga workshops, shaman workshops, A Course in Miracles, and more). The celebration that really blew me away was a marriage proposal from a man who is nothing short of "Love on Two Feet" and a wonderful family reunion. I was living a Technicolor life and loving every minute of it. It was clear to me during this time that "All you really need is Love!"

Humility!

The fall brought many challenges at work with the intense review of our doctoral program along with major course redesign, and challenging national professional association volunteer assignments; all good stuff but challenging nonetheless. Further challenges came when Garrison and I became un-engaged. I also experienced what now appears to have been a major episode of my disease (triggered by some nasty ovarian cysts), which left me literally without my legs and limited arm movement, that all obviously brought me to my knees literally and figuratively. While recovery is going quite well (thanks to all of you), I cancelled five professional trips, something I have never had to face prior. This time taught me lessons of forgiveness, not lessons in how to forgive others for that was not necessary in any of this. Rather, I learned lessons about practicing forgiving myself for the role my ego played in creating so much despair in my life. Louise Hay's[8] quote, "The road to freedom is through the doorway of forgiveness [of self]" makes so much sense to me now.

Surrender!

The winter comes and with it comes renewed strength. I still believe that all we need is love and that love is all there truly is, for everything else is just a cry for love (ACIM). I also believe that as Arnaud Desjardins[9] teaches, "We can not reach love without immense gratitude in our hearts." I am grateful for everything that I experienced this year for without it, I would not be in this place of peace today. Finally, the saying I see all around San Diego County that "Jesus is the reason for the season" helps me to remember that we all hold God within us. Whatever your religion, spirituality, or non-religion, we each already hold the gifts of love, light, peace, and joy within us already. Now, all we need to do is surrender to that power within us and allow ourselves to re-awaken to all the possibilities that are well within our reach.

Wishing you the power to surrender so as to be light, love, joy, and peace in the way that only you are to be.

Lots of love,

Marilee

As I placed the final edits on my letter, I looked up to see if Donita had returned from hiding in the bathroom. Apparently, she was going to wait until the handsome guy, who I now just noticed at the front of the coffee counter line, the guy that she had been expressing an interest in for almost three months, left the building. I giggled to myself. He had

---

8   Louise Hay. *You Can Heal Your Life*. Carlsbad, CA: Hay House Publishing, 1999.

9   Arnaud Desjardins. *Toward the Fullness of Life: The Fullness of Love*. Hohm Press. 1995.

just ordered an extra large specialty drink. Her exit from her bathroom-hiding place may take a while, I thought. I may have to pull the fire alarm to get her out of there.

Returning to my letter, I reread it. Well, that was as summarized of a summary as I could write. I wanted to share much more. However, what was too much to share? Was this already too much to share? My friends teased me for living my life aloud. They further teased me for having a laugh that matched my living style, always recognizable from the farthest distances. I smiled at recalling all their jokes about me and looked up once more. No sign of Donita, and therefore, no coffee refill.

Returning to my thoughts, I looked around the coffee house. It was the morning of December 24. There was a mixture of folks in the coffee house; I was surprised how packed it was. I saw romantic couples nuzzling and kissing, single folks looking way too preoccupied at and a bit annoyed by the couples, harried shoppers glancing down nervously at their watches, and others, just hanging out, like I was doing.

I smiled, warmed by the scene, and glanced back down at my laptop. The cursor had stopped on the word "Surrender." My smile grew even wider. That word held a great deal of meaning to me from this past year. While the word should have had the most meaning from the reoccurrence of the disease and the fun I had saying aloud to myself, "This is not real; what is not real cannot be threatened," as the very handsome firemen wheeled me out of the coffee shop in which I collapsed, another surrender had occurred just recently.

I had been dating a beautiful man. As I was dating him, I was experiencing a great deal of anxiety about our relationship. I had thought that perhaps I was afraid to love again and blah, blah, blah. I found myself weaving another story around why I was anxious. Finally, my fabulous friends reminded me to simply surrender. Had I not surrendered into the relationship and into the place of fully being with this beautiful man, I would not have realized that I was not able to breathe there. He was a beautiful man, but he was not a match for me. I couldn't breathe when I was with him.

Surrender is good; it is great, even when it might be scary. I realized that once I surrendered, I could remove myself as gracefully from the place of not being able to breathe as easily as I could move into child's pose during yoga when I found that I was not breathing in a more difficult asana. Surrender is good. In surrendering, I found that I was not afraid to fall in love again; rather I feared my ability to forgive myself should something go awry in the relationship. I realized I didn't need to tell a story around that. I just needed to see it for what it was, allowing this beautiful man to go his own way and me to go my own way. I needed to surrender into that decision and just breathe.

A laugh I knew and cherished rang in my ears and pulled me from my thoughts. It was Donita. She had come out of her bathroom hiding place and was chatting with the guy she had been admiring from afar for weeks. She was glowingly engaged in the conversation. I watched their courtship dance for a while. The smile on my face was warming my entire body. I looked down to edit my letter once more, but I didn't get very far. Donita and her prince charming were at my table. Donita let me know that they would be chatting for a while longer. She wanted to make sure I was okay by myself. I giggled aloud, reassuring her that I was fine. I watched as they strolled toward a booth, casually and purposefully bumping into each other.

I love it, I thought to myself. Clearly she surrendered. Looking down at my watch, I realized that if I shut down my computer now, I wouldn't have to rush to the next yoga class. Giggling aloud even more, I announced to anyone who would hear, "I surrendered and I no longer have to rush to yoga."

As I packed up my laptop to make my way to yoga class, a text from one of my dear friends came in. I stopped for a moment to read it. My friend was wishing me a merry Christmas and was asking me whether I had answered my calling this year. The words resonated within me, and I felt my body shake as the message settled into my soul. Stepping back for a moment to catch my breath, I sat back down in my booth to call him. He picked up right away.

"Hey Reyal," I spoke into the phone rather excitedly, barely giving him time to even breathe, let alone actually answer. "I just got your text and I had to call." As we exchanged brief Christmas greetings and updates on our lives, I moved to ask him about the question he had posted. I specifically asked him why he had sent it and what it had meant.

He explained to me that he felt that people were called to their spiritual awakening. He explained that you can choose a career, but when you are called to awaken, you either respond or you don't. If you respond, the path appears before you one step at a time. He explained that the path of a calling is revealed to you as you follow it, versus a career that you choose where you plan your path and set your goals. He wanted to know if I had finally answered my calling.

I felt like an idiot but I had to admit to him that I had no idea how to answer his question.

"Geez, Reyal, the most I know is that I responded to your text by calling you. Does that count?"

I thought I was funnier than ever with that one. Reyal, however, didn't laugh. I had no real answer for him. I wasn't even sure I understood the question. As I thanked him for his loving concern, his challenging question, and his beautiful time, I hung up the phone to realize that now, I was going to have to rush to get to yoga; it was the last class of the day because of the holiday schedule. If I missed this one, I would have to wait until the twenty-sixth for the next class.

Pausing for a moment to pray my ACIM prayer, "Where would you have me go? What would you have me do? And what would you have me say and to whom?" I got the sense that it was simply time to go home. There was no need to rush to yoga; there was no need for a yoga "fix," as Philip Urso[10] so cleverly paints the picture of it in our need to calm down through meditation and yoga as if it were a pill. It was simply time to go home, and I got this weird sense that it was time to answer my calling.

As I drove home, feeling reaffirmed by surrendering to the need to NOT rush to yoga, I found myself thinking about Reyal's text. *Have*

10   Philip Urso. Yoga=Heroin, *Elephant Journal*, www.elephantjournal.com/2011/01/yoga-heroin/

I answered my calling? I have a job, no, a profession. I have a profession that I love. I adore my students, the people with whom I work, and I feel so blessed to live in San Diego. Even though I often feel as if I am not making any difference at all, the belief that I am and the smiles on students' faces as a light goes on inside them is richly rewarding and motivating. So, how is this profession not a calling? Surely no one goes into education for the money!

Have I said yes to my calling already? Or is there something I am missing? Unloading my yoga bag onto my living room floor, I plopped onto the floor, feeling rather burdened. I knew I was missing a lesson in all of this. I opened up my laptop to reread my holiday letter. The word "surrender" caught my attention again. I reviewed the lessons I had learned that year, and I summarized them again by admitting that in surrendering to the messages that my mind, body, heart, and soul were conveying, I no longer felt a need to rush to yoga. That was awesome; a huge celebration. Now, perhaps it was time to surrender to something else. Do I surrender to my profession? Or do I surrender to a call? If the latter, what call? From whom? When? And how? I glanced down at my Blackberry as if expecting a phone call from God, and I laughed heartily to myself at the thought of it all.

Placing my Blackberry aside, I leaned toward my yoga bag, pulled my mat from it, and unrolled it across the floor. I arranged myself upon it so as to have my head underneath the manger scene that was displayed on the coffee table and my feet underneath the Christmas tree. I laid down in Savasana, sweet surrender pose.

"The answer to how is yes?" I said aloud to myself as I lay on my living room floor. "How do I stop rushing to yoga? Yes! Am I ready to answer my call, whatever it may be or wherever it may lead? Yes!"

As I drifted off into prayers of gratitude, my phone rang. I had forgotten to shut it off. Sitting up so quickly I almost knocked my head on the coffee table, I laughed as I reached for the phone. Maybe it is God calling with some sort of explanation about my calling. However, most likely, it was my parents. I used to think they (God and my parents) were one and the same when I was little, and now I understood that to be true. However, now I understood it in a different way. Laughing to myself even more at the thought of all of this, I picked up the phone. It was another dear friend.

"Marilee," I heard Nathaniel's voice. "I know you will think this crazy but I was given a name of a person that you must meet. Her name is Lori. Can you meet with her within the week?"

I smiled to myself. The usual me would have asked seventeen more questions before determining whether I would meet with this woman named Lori or not. However, today, still in surrender mode, I simply took down the name and number and affirmed to Nathaniel that I would call her right away.

After Nathaniel and I chatted a little bit longer about our usual nothing in particular, I phoned Lori. I assumed she would be busy with holiday preparations, and it would most likely take two weeks before we even connected. However, it only took one ring. Lori picked up the phone immediately.

"Lori?" I sheepishly said very surprised to be talking to a live voice.

"Yes," the reluctant voice responded.

"This may sound crazy, but I was told to call you. My name is Marilee. I understand I am supposed to meet you." I felt as if I was hanging onto the edge of a cliff, holding my breathe, waiting for the silence to be filled. *What am I doing calling someone I don't know for a reason of which I have no idea?*

The silence evaporated and was replaced with a warm and loving voice.

"Marilee, ah yes. I have been expecting your phone call."

I was immediately relieved by the life and love I sensed in Lori's voice. We spoke for a while longer. I had no idea why I was to meet her but I made arrangements to do so. As I hung up the phone, tears began to flow down my cheeks. They were the tears of sweet surrender.

There is a reason that every yoga practice ends in the same asana. I now understand. I surrendered, and I no longer rush to yoga. I surrendered and said yes to answering a call to which I have no idea of where I am going. This will all be another fun adventure; one that I trust will take me further into living in authenticity.

ABOUT THE AUTHOR

Marilee J. Bresciani is a professor of postsecondary education at San Diego State University. She has no expertise on the subject matter in this book, except that she has simply lived the life written about in this book and is still learning the lessons she shares. Her now more than twenty-four years of professional work has been committed to changing the way that America talks about quality of higher education. In order to keep from going crazy about trying to get the American public to care about what students are actually learning and how they are developing, rather than care about other indicators that have nothing to do with that, she has sought out yoga and meditation. Marilee is currently undergoing yoga teacher training through the Baron Baptiste Power Yoga Institute. Marilee's mantra is "I teach what I need to learn."

RESOURCES

This section requires a bit of introduction. I have compiled this section because these resources have helped me along my journey; moving me from not having a clue about how to grow into my authenticity to at least being able to converse about it. The resources listed here, as well as all the angels who have touched my soul along this journey thus far, have been priceless.

My spiritual introduction and therefore, my introduction to begin questioning whether I was living the life I was called to live came from two beautiful souls who were attending the same conference that I was in Costa Rica. The timing of the meeting was perfect, as my second divorce was only one month from being finalized. Having failed at a second marriage, I was beside myself with confusion about where my meaning making resided. Other than my academic work, which I love greatly, I didn't know what anything else was really about, and I wasn't sure how to move in any world other than the academic one. I am so grateful to these two souls for simply asking me questions and allowing me to ask questions in return. The inquiry process (simply asking questions in a manner that opens up possibilities, rather than closing off possibilities) opened the door to a new experience, one that led me to redefine how I make meaning.

Spiritual inquiry is the best way to describe my journey thus far. This section, similar to this book, seeks not to establish my voice as authority, but rather to share with others, from a place of simple daily experiences and inquiry. My hope is that the application of inquiry on daily life will allow others to discover their paths to their own authentic way of being—to their authentic selves.

The first set of resources I share are those that my sister, Elizabeth, shared with me when I first became sick and was losing the use of my legs. I used to run to rid myself of stress. No longer having the ability to run, I was working myself into a worried frenzy. I wasn't finding my religion to be of aid in this moment. So my sister suggested I read the following Thich Nhat Hanh books, published by Bantam. I highly recommend them because they helped me understand that religion can be spiritual yet the way I had been practicing religion lacked the presence of spirit. I was doing what I thought I should instead of questioning whether what I was doing was resonating with who I was designed to be. The following books helped me get started with some inquiry into spiritual practices that I could either adopt or not adopt.

Living Christ: Living Buddha
Peace Is Every Step
The Art of Power
Taming the Tiger Within
True Love
A Guide to Walking Meditation

My friend, Jan, introduced me to yoga and meditation. By the time I finally got around to taking her up on the offer, I was in too much pain from my disease; however, her loving prodding never left me, and as explained in this book, the introduction to yoga on the mat and off the mat opened up inquiry and therefore possibilities I never imagined.

Yoga has become so popular today, yet it is also, in my opinion, often misunderstood. In this quick overview, I share more about what yoga is not, rather than what it is. For example, yoga is not intended to be a religion, even though the philosophy of yoga is present in Hinduism, Buddhism, and Jainism. To illustrate, I recently mentioned to one of my Christian students, "When you do yoga, you are not praying to a Hindu god, unless you want to pray to a Hindu god. However, given your religion, you may prefer to pray to your Jesus or the father of your Jesus. Or you may choose not to pray at all. Yoga doesn't really care if you pray while you are on or off your mat. That is entirely up to you.

I understand that yoga, which originated in India, is a uniting of the mind, body, and spirit through several asanas. "Asana" is a Sanskrit word used to name several types of body positions intended primarily to improve flexibility, vitality, and overall well-being. In addition, yoga is intended to promote one's ability to remain in seated meditation for extended periods, a pretty handy benefit if your mind and your body tend to be a bit overactive as mine do.

Some of the asanas referred to in this book indicate child's pose (Sanskrit = Blasana), which is basically a fetal pose on the floor, sitting back on your heels with your forehead to the ground, arms by your sides or arms stretched out in front of you. Another is Savasana (Sanskrit name) or corpse pose. I prefer to call it surrender; it sounds happier. Here, you lie on your back, arms at your side, and you simply rest. The idea is to end each yoga practice in Savasana in order to seal in your practice, seal in your learning, seal in your awakenings, and provide one last opportunity to unite mind, body, and spirit in rest as well as rejuvenation. This pose, in my opinion, fully prepares me for meditation.

Books that I have found helpful in learning about asanas, what they look like, what they do for you, and how to string them together to form a balanced practice include Baron Baptiste's books published by Fireside from Simon and Schuster. Baronbaptise.com also has DVDs in case you would prefer to watch how this stuff can be integrated into your life versus read about it.

40 Days to Personal Revolution: A Breakthrough Program to Radically Change Your Body and Awaken the Sacred within Your Soul
Journey into Power: How to Sculpt Your Ideal Body, Free Your True Self, and Transform Your Life with Yoga
The Yoga Bootcamp Box: An Interactive Program to Revolutionize Your Life with Yoga

More information can be found also at www.baronbaptiste.com and www.saltpondyoga.com

My friends Cyd, Ralph, and Jan introduced me to meditation practices through their own practices, yoga, and books by Abraham Hicks, Eckart Tolle, and Thich Nhat Hanh. It was Chris Meredith who really helped me to understand the importance of meditating daily. Chris, along with Philip Urso and Baron Baptiste, illustrated all the inquiry and therefore the possibilities that open when I sat in silence.

To me, meditation is a quieting of the mind by focusing on my breathing. In other words, for twenty to thirty minutes each day, I sit upright or lie on my back and focus on my breathing. Yup, that is it. I spend twenty to thirty minutes a day focusing on my inhale and exhale. As thoughts come up (and they always do), I practice observing thoughts that arise, as I would observe a bird in flight. So, every time a thought interrupts my meditation, I see it as a bird passing through my meditation. I observe the bird but I choose not to speak to it. To an observer, my practice of meditation might look something like this:

Inhale, exhale, inhale, exhale. Here comes a bird, oh, look at the bird. Oh, there it goes. Inhale, exhale, inhale, exhale. Here comes another bird. Hi birdie. Hey, I wonder if this one will drop something on my head. No wait, don't think about what the bird will do, don't talk to the bird, just watch it fly by. Okay. Bye bird. Inhale. Exhale. Inhale. Exhale.

More information on deepening your meditation practice can be found in the Thich Nhat Hanh books or by e-mailing Chris Meredith at cheshireman22@directv.net

My friend Danny introduced me to A Course in Miracles (ACIM) (www.acim.org) through Philip Urso's Salt Pond Yoga Studio and ACIM podcasts (www.saltpondyoga.com). These podcasts and readings were brought to life for me further through Drew, who organized the North Park Course in Miracles Meet-up Group. The ACIM discussion group at Unity Church in San Diego has also been instrumental in helping me apply the ACIM principles to my moment-to-moment life.

A Course in Miracles is not a religion. To me, it is a way of being and it is a great inquiry process into how I think and feel. ACIM doesn't tell me what to do, it asks me to question what I think and do. ACIM illustrates a way to inquire that has the potential to literally retrain the mind to question daily thoughts and therefore, interpret daily circumstances as opportunities to learn how to practice loving thoughts, words, and actions instead of reacting as if I am a victim to those same circumstances. Instead of creating stories out of my egocentric mind, where I am a victim and everyone else is the perpetrator, ACIM empowers me to ask questions about them which moves me from my head into my heart and then I can choose to act out of love, Oneness, joy, and peace. Empowered by the Holy Spirit, or whatever you want to call your God or source power (ACIM doesn't care), I call upon the Holy Spirit to reveal to me the daily opportunities to learn how to be more loving in all ways in all situations. The power of the Holy Spirit also shows me where I need to let something go and reveals to me the Oneness of us all. All I need to do is choose to call upon the Holy Spirit every moment of every day and inquire, when I forget to do that, to simply choose again in the next moment.

I am confident that A Course in Miracles teachings would not have landed so well in my life had I not been prepared for their lessons via other fabulous friends, experiences, and readings such as those that follow:

- The wonderful yoga instructors at Core Power Yoga in San Diego (www.corepoweryoga.com)
- Lori Pettigrew, astrologer, at loripettigrew@gmail.com
- Dr. Charlie Sanders, Lifesource Network Chiropractic, at bodyheals@yahoo.com
- Dr. Adrian Bean at the Healing Point (www.thehealingpoint. com)
- Diana Pepper at Tree Frog Farm (www.treefrogfarm.com)
- Laura Lee, massage therapist (www.bikramyoga.com/ studioDetails.php?id=278)
- Byron Katie's books (www.thework.com/index.php)
- Neale Donald Walsch, Conversations with God books (www.nealedonaldwalsch.com)

- Louise Hay's books (www.louisehay.com)
- Abraham Hicks's teachings (www.abraham-hicks.com/lawofattractionsource/index.php)
- Marianne Williamson's books (www.marianne.com)
- Deepak Chopra's books (www.chopra.com)
- Gary Renard's books (www.garyrenard.com)

Then, there are those awakenings that seem to occur frequently in certain locations; some might call these locations spiritual vortexes (daily places where spiraling spiritual energy facilitates healing, meditation, and prayer). I just like to call them "daily places that seem to be frequent locations for where my awakenings occur." The following are some of those places:

- In thought and conversations at my kitchen counter
- Driving my Jeep Wrangler
- In conversations with Dan, present at the Red Velvet Wine Bar in Little Italy
- Drinking green tea soy lattes with no classic and no foam at the Starbucks in Hillcrest, Camino Del Rio N., and in Point Loma
- On the dance floor of Humphreys Back Stage Live and Patricks II at the Gaslamp
- On walks on Cowles Mountain, Mission Trails Park, San Diego
- Sipping coffee or tea and looking at the ocean at Cantina or Kono's coffee shops, Pacific Beach boardwalk

In summary, these resources are provided in the hopes that they will assist you in creating your own tool kit, your own list of resources to facilitate your own inquiry and your reconnection to your authentic self. I encourage you to share with those you love that which assists you in being present in love and contributing to your awakening to your greatest good. Ask them to coach you daily, moment-by moment.

Create your community where you can love your personal life into a place where you are supported to become all that you can be. Our friends, family, and coworkers can become our greatest teachers if we allow them to do so.

Namaste,

Marilee

For more information, see
http://interwork.sdsu.edu/elip/consultation/index.html

REFERENCES

Baron Baptiste. (2010). *Foundations in Teacher Training Workshop.* Park City, UT. www.baronbaptiste.com

Desjardins, Arnaud. (1995). *Toward the Fullness of Life: The Fullness of Love.* Prescott, AZ: Hohm Press.

Foundation for Inner Peace. (1975). *A Course in Miracles.* www.acim.org

Hay, Louise. (1999). *You Can Heal Your Life.* Carlsbad, CA: Hay House Publishing.

Palmer, Parker J. (2000). *Let Your Life Speak: Listening for the Voice of Vocation.* San Francisco, CA: Jossey Bass Publishing.

Urso, Philip. (January 13, 2011). Yoga=Heroin. *Elephant Journal,* http://www.elephantjournal.com/2011/01/yoga-heroin/

Williamson, Marianne (1992). *A Return to Love: Reflections on the Principles of the Course in Miracles.* New York: HarperCollins.

www.ingramcontent.com/pod-product-compliance
Lightning Source LLC
Chambersburg PA
CBHW051415280526
45785CB00003B/1068